Anesthesia Made Easy:
The Survival Guide to Make Your First Anesthesia Rotation a Success

© 2015 Two Pugs Publishing
All rights reserved.
Alpha.Pug@TwoPugsPublishing.com

ISBN: 978-0-9898401-3-2
eISBN: 978-0-9898401-4-9

Material in this book is for educational purposes only and does not constitute medical advice or create a doctor-patient relationship. The book and the website AnesthesiaMadeEasy.com are intended for medical professionals and students who have formal education in general medicine and have or are in the process of learning the skills necessary to take care of patients during the perioperative period, while under the guidance of a licensed professional experienced in the practice of anesthesiology.

Knowledge and best practices in the field of anesthesiology are constantly changing. As new information is gained through research and clinical experience, it may be appropriate to change treatment and medication therapy. Readers are urged to check the most current information provided in the field of medicine and to review manufacturer information to verify the recommended dose, method and duration of administration, warnings, precautions and contraindications for medications and procedures presented. Some drugs and devices discussed in this book have limited or restricted FDA (Food and Drug Administration) clearance. It is the responsibility of the reader to ascertain the FDA status of each drug or device for use in a clinical setting.

This book is intended as an overview and guide, and is in no means exhaustive in its scope. It is the responsibility of the practitioner to determine dosages and best practices for each patient based on his or her experience and the circumstances of patient treatment. Ultimately, the administration of anesthesia and care of the patient rests on the practitioner.

Care has been taken to confirm that the information presented is correct and is in line with generally accepted practices. That being said, the author, editors, contributors, and publisher are not responsible for errors or omissions of information or for any direct or indirect consequences of the application of information in this book and website AnesthesiaMadeEasy.com. Neither the author, editors, contributors, nor the publisher make any warranty, express or implied, or assume any liability for injury and/or damage to persons or property arising out of or related to any use of the material contained in this book.

Why you need *Anesthesia Made Easy*.

Most introductory anesthesia books are too long and too complex. Where do you begin learning about anesthesia when the basic books are over 800 pages long and weigh four pounds? Even when you do read these books, how will you translate the information into something you can use in the operating room when you are first starting out?

Welcome to *Anesthesia Made Easy*.

I wrote this book to introduce you to anesthesiology. It is part education guide (to teach you the basics of anesthesia) and part survival guide (to teach you how to apply these basics while in the operating room). It includes the basics of anesthesia without getting too far into the weeds and also gives you a practical approach that will get you started moving in the right direction.

When I was chief resident at UT Southwestern Medical Center, I developed a new system on how to train new anesthesia residents titled Vapor Camp. It is a revolutionary way to give interns exposure to the operating room, anesthesia didactics, and simulation scenarios before they are expected to perform on their own. Now, as Vapor Camp approaches its seventh year, I have realized that the program needs a manual: *Anesthesia Made Easy*.

Currently, I train airway rotators, anesthesiologist assistant students, medical students, residents, and fellows in the art and science of anesthesiology through lectures and in the OR.

New anesthesiology students struggle with which book to read and where to start. This book will give you not only a solid foundation upon which to start your career but also organize the information in such a way that you can actually use it.

- If you are doing **anesthesia observations or shadowing** to see if anesthesia is a good fit for you, you should start with chapter 1, "How to Get the Most from Your Anesthesiology Observation." Then read chapter 4, "Anesthesiology Basic Concepts," and chapter 5, "Getting Around in the OR," to learn the culture of the OR — they will bring you a long way.

- If you are **an airway rotator,** concentrate on chapter 19, "Airway Exam and Evaluation," chapter 7, "Basic Anesthesia Pharmacology: Medications," and chapter 24 "Adult Airway Management," chapter 25 "Pediatric Airway Management," and chapter 27 "Rapid Sequence Induction (RSI)."

- If you are on your **first anesthesia rotation**, start at the front of *Anesthesia Made Easy* and work your way through before you start your rotation. This book is meant to be a quick read. Bring the book with you to the operating room and take notes in the notes section. Then when you go home, pull out one of the basic books listed in chapter 34, "Anesthesia Resources," and read up on the topics that you want more information on.

- If you are an **anesthesia tech** or working toward your **anesthesia technologist certification**, this book will give you an introduction to the art and science of anesthesiology. It should give you an overview of what anesthesia is like and should help you see the specialty from a different viewpoint. Start at the front and work your way through to the end. Ask questions and take notes to help you be better at your job. As you prepare for your exam, I have listed some resources for you at AnesthesiaMadeEasy.com.

- If you are **applying to AA or CRNA school**, then read this book cover to cover before you interview. It will give you a working knowledge of the type of training you will receive. It may also help you in your interview process to give you answers to simple questions about anesthesia care.

- If you are **medical school student applying to an anesthesiology residency**, check out my website, AnesthesiaMadeEasy.com, which offers a free e-book, *Getting into Anesthesiology*, to help guide you through the application process.

This is my interpretation of the art and science of anesthesiology as I know it. There are many different ways to safely care for patients under anesthesia. This book is just to get you pointed in the right direction. *Anesthesiology Made Easy* should be your jumping off point; this book will teach you a lot of the "how, " but you will likely need to read other books to learn more of the "why" as you go through your training.

I wish you well as you start your career in anesthesiology.

Jeff Steiner, DO, MBA

Acknowledgments

I want to extend a heartfelt thank you to all my beta readers (listed in alphabetical order below). Without your assistance, I would have published several mistakes, and a few faux pas.

Ty Carl, BS
Eugene Chung, DO
Jana McAlister, MS, MMSc, AA-C
Ryan A Sexton, RN, MSN, CRNA
Jennifer C. Steiner, PA-C
Peter Szmuk, MD
Amy P. Woods, MD

I also want to thank my online team that helped me bring this project to a new level.

Book Cover Design by Daryl Orosco at Designers-Pro™ through 99desgins.com.

Professional Editing Services by Karen Otis through ProofreadingPal.com.

Table of Contents

The following are some of the basic concepts you should strive to understand and explain:

Basic skills you should work toward:

The Thoughts

The Movements

The following are the different types of anesthesia:

Sedation

General Anesthesia (GA)

Regional Anesthesia (RA)

Combining the Different Types of Anesthesia Techniques

The Four Stages of Anesthesia

Comparing Potency of Anesthesia Medications – MAC

Anesthesiology and Flying a Plane

How the Gases/Vapors Work

Medical Gases

Anesthesia Vapors

Anesthesia Pharmacology Introduction

Five things to check before giving the medications:

IV Fluids and Blood

Crystalloid Fluids

Colloid Fluids

Blood Products

Fluid Replacement

1. Getting the Most from Your Anesthesiology Observation

A career in anesthesia is not for everyone. Observing anesthesia the first time can be overwhelming. There are many moving parts in the operating room and several transitions that patients go through. The anesthesia team is responsible for not only the operative period (while in the OR) but also the preoperative care (to make sure the patient is "ready" for surgery) and postoperative care (to make sure the patient successfully transitions from the OR to the postanesthesia care unit [PACU] or intensive care unit [ICU]). Along with taking care of patients, there are also time constraints placed on the whole OR team. You will see different members of the anesthesia and OR teams working together to bring the patient safely through the perioperative period. Keep a "situational awareness" as to what is going on in the OR. There will be times that the anesthesiologist, anesthesia resident/fellow, or anesthesia provider (anesthesiologist assistant [AA] or certified registered nurse anesthetist [CRNA][1]) will not have time to talk with you. Don't take it personally. If things are tense, write down your question to ask later. Talking with the members of the anesthesia team will help you to learn about the practice of anesthesia and what they like and do not like about a career in anesthesia.

Before you start your observation, read chapter 4, "Anesthesiology Basic Concepts," and chapter 5, "Getting

---

[1] Throughout this book, I have ordered anesthesiologist assistant (AA) or certified registered nurse anesthetist (CRNA) alphabetically. AA is a relatively new profession compared to CRNA.

Around in the OR," to get a framework of what you will be seeing. While you are on your observational experience, pick a few things a day to learn about. Read about them in the corresponding chapters in this book, and go to the OR with a focus on those topics for the day. Then, the next day, choose some different topics and go from there. This is your time to explore anesthesia, so make the most of it. Be engaged, and try to get a feel for what a career would be like.

2. What You Should Learn on Your First Anesthesiology Rotation

      Try to read this book from cover to cover before you start your rotation. The first time you read about anesthesiology, you will not understand everything and that is all right. After you have started your rotation, read through it again, and things will start to make more sense.

      Because anesthesiology is a specialty of *thinking* and *doing*, it will take seeing the anesthesia processes in action for some concepts to make sense. With so much new information to learn, anesthesiology can be overwhelming. Pick one or two things a day to concentrate on and learn them.

The following are some of the basic concepts you should strive to understand and explain:

- The four components of general anesthesia (GA). (ch. 4: "Anesthesiology Basic Concepts")

- The concept of minimal alveolar concentration (MAC). (ch. 4: "Anesthesiology Basic Concepts")

- The stages of anesthesia and what they mean. (ch. 4: "Anesthesiology Basic Concepts")

- Vapor choices and selection (ch. 6: "Basic Anesthesia Pharmacology: Gases and Vapors")

- Common medications and their selection (ch. 7: "Basic Anesthesia Pharmacology: Medications")

Basic skills you should work toward:

- How to complete a basic machine check (ch. 21: "Anesthesia Machine and Monitors")
- The basic room setup (ch. 22: "Setting Up Your Room")
- How to draw up drugs (ch. 22: "Setting Up Your Room")
- Know which drugs need to be diluted (ch. 12: "Autonomic Nervous System Medications")
- How to mask, place an laryngeal mask airway (LMA), and intubate an adult patient (ch. 24: "Adult Airway Management")
- How to set up an IV bag (have someone show you how)
- How to start an IV (have someone show you how)

3. How to Study Anesthesiology

Anesthesiology has a good balance between both thoughts and movements.

The Thoughts

One of the best ways to learn anesthesiology is to read about a subject, go see it in the OR, and then read again about what you saw in the OR. Keep this guide handy in the OR for quick references and note-taking.

When you read about anesthesia, there will be things that will not make sense. (The machine check comes to mind.) That's OK. Read through the book according to the guide, then go into the OR and watch it in action. After seeing anesthesiology *in action*, the reading will make a lot more sense. To understand the rationale behind what we do, you need to understand the concepts.

The Movements

Anesthesiology is a procedure-heavy specialty. We do a large number of high-risk, invasive procedures. We have low complication rates because we respect the patient and we respect the procedure. Take time to understand what you are doing. Remember you are doing procedures on real patients who have entrusted their care to the anesthesia team. **Never view your time as practicing on patients**. Respect that and respect your patients.

My best advice to you comes from the US Navy SEALS: "Slow is smooth … smooth is fast."

In the beginning of your training, understand the mechanics (where to put the tip of the laryngoscope blade, the tip of the needle, etc.) and don't rush through the procedure in an effort to do it quickly. Speed will come later. Now is the time to learn the proper technique. With the proper technique ingrained in your training, you will be safer, quicker, and look more confident.

Slow is smooth … smooth is fast.

4. Anesthesiology Basic Concepts

The following are the different types of anesthesia:

Sedation

This is the process of providing medications to induce hypnosis and decrease pain and anxiety.

The following are the sedation levels as described by the American Society of Anesthesiologists (ASA):

- Minimal Sedation (Anxiolysis) – "Normal response to verbal stimulation."
- Moderate Sedation (Conscious Sedation) – "Purposeful response to verbal or tactile stimulation."
- Deep Sedation – "Purposeful response after repeated or painful stimulation."
- General Anesthesia (Obtunded) – "Unarousable even with painful stimulus."

General Anesthesia (GA)

- This is the process of making the patient insensible to surgical stimulus.
- Five things are combined to provide GA
    1. anxiolysis – usually administered prior to the procedure
    2. amnesia
    3. hypnosis – the continuum of sedation (as described above)
    4. pain control (analgesia)
    5. chemical paralysis (also known as muscle relaxation)

Regional Anesthesia (RA)

- This technique places local anesthesia next to nerves to "numb" them to pain. RA can be used as a sole anesthetic or in combination with sedation or GA to keep the patient comfortable during surgery and/or for postoperative pain control.

There are two broad categories of regional anesthesia:

1. **Neuraxial**
   - Spinal or epidural anesthesia/analgesia
   - Provides pain relief to a large region of the body
2. **Peripheral nerve blocks**
   - Blocks a distribution of a nerve or a group of related nerves
   - Provides pain relief to an extremity or smaller region of the body

Combining the Different Types of Anesthesia Techniques

All these techniques can be used in various combinations to provide an anesthetic plan that is tailored for the patient. Sometimes conditions change and the anesthetic plan needs to be modified as well. For example, sedation may not be enough to keep the patient safe and comfortable; therefore, GA may need to be initiated.

The Four Stages of Anesthesia

General anesthesia can be described as having multiple stages. These stages were first described with ether and are sometimes called the "ether planes."

Stage 1 – Analgesia

- The patient becomes sedated.

Stage 2 – Excitation

- There is an increase in heart rate (HR) and blood pressure (BP).
- Patient may become combative as he or she goes through this stage.

Stage 3 – Surgical Anesthesia

- The HR and BP begin to return to baseline.
- The patient is "deep" enough for surgery to begin.

Stage 4 – Coma

- The patient's vital signs collapse.

Stages of Anesthesia Concepts

With each increase in stage, you will see an escalation in the depth of anesthesia. When patients have anesthesia induced by inhaling anesthesia medication through an anesthesia machine, you will see the patient go through stage 1 and through stage 2 (hopefully briefly) to stage 3. (We call this a mask induction.) When an IV induction is preformed, the onset of GA is so fast you will not see the patient go through stage 2. You will observe the patient go from awake through stage 1 and directly to stage 3.

When patients wake up from the anesthetic, you will see them go in reverse order from stage 3 through stage 2 to stage 1 and then awake. It is during the transition through stage 2 that "waking up" from anesthesia can be dangerous. This is because the patients may move and act as if they are awake, but they are in fact still heavily sedated. It is also during this time that the patient may vomit or retch, and therefore, extubating the patient during this time can lead to aspiration (stomach contents going into the lungs) or laryngospasm (when the vocal cords and attached structures close). Both of these events can lead to serious consequences.

Comparing Potency of Anesthesia Medications – MAC

Minimal alveolar concentration (MAC) is a way to compare the strengths, or potency, of anesthesia vapors and other medications to have a sense of how much anesthesia someone is getting. MAC is a helpful, albeit somewhat confusing, concept for you to understand. Each vapor and gas has a MAC associated with it. For example, 1 MAC of sevoflurane is 1.8, whereas the MAC of desflurane is about 6.6. The MAC for each vapor and gas has been determined and is something that can be looked up (see Table 1).

Table 1 Comparison of Anesthesia Vapors				
Anesthetic Vapor	1 MAC %	Minimal Fresh Gas Flows	Pros	Cons
isoflurane	1.17	1 L/m	Cardio-protective	slow wake up
sevoflurane	1.85	2 L/m	good for mask induction / least pungent	renal failure in rats with low gas flow
desflurane	6.6	1 L/m	good for obese patients	irritating for smokers and asthmatics

Four Concepts to Know about MAC

1.   **MAC works on a continuum:**
- 1 MAC is the amount of medication needed so that 50% of patients will not move to painful stimuli. 1.3 MAC is needed for 99% of patients not to move under painful stimuli. Each vapor has its own concentration equivalent to 1 MAC. (See ch. 6, "Basic Anesthesia Pharmacology: Vapors and Gases.")
- MAC awake = 0.3 MAC
- MAC recall = 0.7 MAC

2. **MAC is additive:**
    - If you add 0.5 MAC of a gas (50% nitrous oxide) to 0.5 MAC of a vapor (~1% sevoflurane), you will have the equivalent of about 1 MAC of the total gas.
3. **MAC can be affected by the patient's current conditions:**
    - MAC values were developed by utilizing healthy 40 year olds who were not receiving other medications. A patient's age and other health conditions can increase or decrease MAC requirements.
    - Some medications, such as propofol, opioids, and acute alcohol, decrease a patient's vapor MAC requirement.
    - Other medications, such as cocaine, ephedrine, and chronic alcohol, require an increase in vapor MAC to achieve the same affect.
4. **MAC is displayed on most modern anesthesia monitors:**
    - The MAC displayed will be calculated from the gases and vapors that are currently being used.
    - This information is a helpful guide for you as you are learning how much anesthesia vapors and gas to give.

Anesthesiology and Flying a Plane

The practice of anesthesia is often compared to flying a plane — both take specialized training, both are relatively safe (but can have times of true danger), and both follow a similar progression of events. When flying a plane, most problems occur during takeoff and landing.

Similarly, in anesthesia, most problems occur when the patient is going to sleep and waking up. Although flying a plane is commonly associated with air travel, it is just as important that the plane is ready to fly and is safely escorted to and from the terminal to the landing strip.

Anesthesia encompasses the transition of safe patient care throughout the perioperative period. Perioperative care consists of

- preoperative care (before surgery),
- intraoperative care (during surgery), and
- postoperative care (after surgery).

Preoperative (Getting the Patient Ready for Surgery)

- Anesthesia history and physical (H&P)

- Making sure the patient is at his or her best health for the planed surgery
  (This may mean that the patient's home medication regimen be "tuned up" before having surgery).

- Obtaining IV access or invasive monitors

- Preoperative anxiolysis

Intraoperative (Induction of Anesthesia — Flight Takeoff)

- Inducing anesthesia

- Securing the airway

- Positioning the patient

- Obtaining further monitoring, as needed.

Intraoperative (Maintaining Anesthesia — Cruising at Altitude)

- Continuing to keep the patient comfortable

- Maintaining the anesthesia with vapor, pain control, and muscle relaxation

- Remaining vigilant in keeping the patient safe

Intraoperative (Waking Up—Landing the Plane)

- Titrating the medication to wake up the patient at the end of the case
- Reversing chemical paralytics
- Removing the endotracheal tube or supraglottic device when it is safe to do so
- Bringing the patient to the post-anesthesia care unit

Postoperative Care (Escorting the Plane to the Terminal)

- After surgery, we continue to take care of patients until they have recovered from anesthesia.
- Patients are brought to either
  - the post-anesthesia care unit (PACU) or
  - the intensive care unit (ICU).
- While in both locations, patients have their vital signs, pain, nausea and vomiting, and other medical issues managed.

5. Getting Around in the OR

As with most environments, the operating room (OR) has its own set of cultures and norms. If you have been in the OR before, this chapter should be a quick read for you. You are on this airway or anesthesia rotation as part of the anesthesia care team.

Within the OR environment, remember you are a guest in a new culture. You are joining a culture that has history and rites of passage and that places trust at the forefront. As an "outsider" you will want to do a few things to ensure you start off on the right footing.

Situational awareness is key to a successful experience.

The anesthesia team members may include the following:

- Anesthesiologist
  - A physician who has completed his or her anesthesiology training.
- Anesthesia Resident
  - A physician who is training in anesthesiology.
- Anesthesia Fellow
  - A physician who is doing advanced training in anesthesiology after his or her residency.
- Anesthesiologist Assistant (AA)
  - A medical professional who has had specialized training in anesthesia.
- Certified Nurse Anesthetist (CRNA)
  - An advanced practice nurse who has had specialized training in anesthesia.

- Anesthesia Technician
  - A technician who assists the anesthesia team in room turnover, maintaining equipment and supplies, and providing an extra hand.
- Students and Observers

The OR team members:

- Surgeon
  - The physician in charge of the operation
- Nurse Circulator
  - The nurse who assists with patient care but is not scrubbed in the case.
- Scrub Nurse
  - A nurse who is scrubbed in the case and assists the surgeon.
- Scrub Tech or First Assist
  - A technician who is scrubbed in the case and assists the surgeon.
- Medical Students/Nursing Students/Observers

Anesthesiology Relationship Dynamics

It takes a team of physicians, nurses, operating room techs, anesthesia techs, housekeeping, and administrators to keep the OR going. Treat everyone with respect.

The anesthesia team can be made up of attending anesthesiologists by themselves or with AAs, CRNAs, anesthesiology residents/fellows, and residents and fellows from other specialties. Trainees are also involved in this dynamic and can be residents, medical school students, or AA/CRNA students

<u>The anesthesiology team has three patients: the patient on the table, the surgeon, and the OR team.</u>

You're Not the Boss of Me . . . or Maybe You Are

Most anesthesiologists work for a surgeon. The anesthesia team is there as a consulting service to support the surgeon. They may not be directly employed by him or her, but they do work for the surgeon. Being obnoxious, loud, or inattentive or being rude to the nurses, scrubs, or others, as well as texting on your phone or complaining about the length of the surgery, does not earn you any favors with the surgeon. This is especially true for observers and trainees.

You and your surgeon have a symbiotic relationship. He or she needs you to operate, and you need him or her to bring you cases. Without your surgeons, you would be working in critical care, pain clinics, or on the wards. (Oh, please no.)
This is one of the most important relationships to learn how to manage because it is vital for a successful, long-term career.

As you go through your training, see how surgeons respond to the different anesthesia team members who work with you. Build good relationships with your surgeons, and they will take care of you.

Basic Interactions

Remember that you are a guest. You are working to make a good impression. Those who fit in well, get to do more.

- Listen twice as much as you talk
- Learn to develop a situational awareness

- If things are not going well for the anesthesia/surgical team, try to keep your questions to a minimum.

- Every room and every team has a little different dynamic.

    - Until you know exactly what is going on, try to be very observant.

    - Pay attention to the culture of the room.

- There will be some rooms where there is a lot of talking going on and others where it is dead quiet.

- Be mindful of how you walk through the OR environment.

    - Don't walk too close to the surgical instruments tables and be careful not to touch the surgeon or scrub tech so that you don't contaminate them.

Working in the Operating Room Environment

- Keep your anesthesia area clean.

    - Don't throw discarded equipment or syringe wrappers on the floor. (I learned this the hard way from Marilyn and Al in the burn room at Parkland. I love you guys.)

Going into the OR for the First Time

When you first go into a room, avoid all the surgical instruments and equipment. The quickest way to get tossed from the OR is to contaminate any of the sterile equipment or personnel. (The sterile equipment is usually laid out on tables covered with a large drape or on surgical stands.)

When you first go into the OR, do the following:

1. Introduce yourself to the circulating nurse.
2. Find the members of the anesthesia team and introduce yourself to them as well.
3. Take a look at the anesthesia setup.

   - Where is the drug cart?
   - Where is the anesthesia machine?
   - What is laid out on the anesthesia machine?
   - Don't touch anything on the anesthesia cart. Nothing gets us edgy like someone touching our medications or equipment.

4. If a case is currently going when you arrive in the operating room, look around and ask yourself the following questions:

   - Are there gases flowing?
   - Is there a vaporizer turned on?
   - Find the monitor and figure out where all the vital signs are displayed on the monitor.

     - Electrocardiograph ECG (usually at the top of the screen)
     - Heart rate
     - Pulse oximetry
     - Blood pressure (and the last time it was taken)
     - End title CO_2 (EtCO2)
     - Temperature

- Are the vapors displayed? If so, how much vapor is the patient receiving?
- Some monitors will display the MAC

For those of you who have been in the OR before, this chapter should have been a quick read. Now we will get on with some of the foundational knowledge that will help you as you go through your anesthesiology rotation.

6. Basic Anesthesia Pharmacology: Vapors and Gases

Anesthesia vapors are one of the few medications that are used exclusively in the practice of anesthesiology. Our vapors come in a liquid form that is placed into agent-specific vaporizers. These vaporizers are attached to anesthesia machines that allow for gases (air, oxygen, and nitrous oxide) to pass through the vaporizer and turn the liquid anesthesia medications into a vapor that is then carried to the patient within the anesthesia breathing circuit.

How the Gases/Vapors Work

The gases flow to the anesthesia machine from the pipeline or cylinder, go through the flow meters, go through the vaporizer and carry the vapor to the inspiratory arm of the machine where it goes to the patient.

Once in the patient, the gas/vapor goes to the lungs, and to the blood, to the brain (as well as muscle, bone, and fat) to put the patient asleep. The gas/vapor then leaves the brain, through the blood, to the lung, and is exhaled from the patient. As long as you are delivering a constant supply of vapor, the patient will remain asleep. Some of the gas/vapor is metabolized, but most is "blown off" by the patient, and this is what allows the patient to wake up when the level is low enough.

Medical Gases

- Air – medical grade air (yellow hose)
- Oxygen (O2) – medical grade pure oxygen (green hose)
- Nitrous Oxide (N2O) – also known as laughing gas (blue hose)

- commonly used in dental offices for sedation
- Waste Gases – those gases that are taken away from the machine (white hose)

Anesthesia Vapors

There are three common anesthesia vapors used extensively worldwide:

- Isoflourane (Iso)
- Sevoflurane (Sevo)
- Desflurane (Des)

The unique properties of each vapor determine which one we use. The two main properties that dictate their use are solubility and pungency.

Solubility:

The more soluble a vapor, the longer it will take to come and go from the patient and the longer it will take for the patient to go to sleep and to wake up. (Solubility of vapors—from most soluble to least soluble—Iso > Sevo > Des.) Therefore, Iso takes the longest to wake up from due to the relative large solubility, and likewise, Des is the shortest to wake up from due to its relative insolubility. The solubility of isoflurane makes it an ideal choice for patients who will remain intubated, and historically, it has been used in cardiac patients because it is hemodynamically stable. The insolubility of Des also makes it advantageous for patients who are overweight because they tend to wake up faster as compared to obese patients who are given Iso or Sevo.

Pungency:

The least pungent vapor is Sevo, and it is exclusively used for mask inductions in children in the United States. Des tends to be the most pungent and can be an airway irritant. (This fact is important to remember when using it with patients who smoke or have asthma.)

How do you measure the delivery of the vapor?

The amount of anesthesia vapor given to patients is measured in percentages (see Table 6-1). Each vapor has its own vaporizer with a dial on top with the percentage labeled on it.

To start the flow of a vapor, squeeze the top of the dial to unlock it and turn the dial counterclockwise to deliver the vapor. We often say we "dialed up" the vapor, which means we turned it on or increased the percentage of vapor delivered.

How do you change the amount of vapor going to the patient?

The depth of anesthesia can be changed faster with

1. increased gas flows,
2. increased tidal volumes,
3. increased percentage of vapor, or
4. second gas effect.
    - The second gas effect is discussed a lot in pharmacology books. The concept is that when N2O is used, it diffuses from the lung alveoli into the blood faster than the vapor, which concentrates the vapor left in the lungs.
    - This second gas effect is probably not clinically relevant.

Table 1 Comparison of Anesthesia Vapors				
Anesthetic Vapor	$\frac{1}{MAC}$ %	Minimal Fresh Gas Flows	Pros	Cons
isoflurane	1.17	1 L/m	Cardio-protective	slow wake up
sevoflurane	1.85	2 L/m	good for mask induction / least pungent	renal failure in rats with low gas flow
desflurane	6.6	1 L/m	good for obese patients	irritating for smokers and asthmatics

7. Basic Anesthesia Pharmacology: Medications

Anesthesia Pharmacology Introduction

There are whole textbooks written on the pharmacology we use in anesthesiology. In an effort to keep this section readable and at a reasonable length, I have decided to include the most common medications you will encounter. In my opinion, having pages upon pages of vapors and medications that are not widely used (or in some cases not even produced anymore) is of little value to you when you are just starting in anesthesiology.

For further pharmacology reading, there are some great chapters in *Basics of Anesthesia* by Drs. Miller and Pardo and *Morgan and Mikhail's Clinical Anesthesiology* by Drs. Butterworth, Mackey, and Wasnick that can help you grasp the concepts of pharmacology. A great review book for basic pharmacology is *Lippincott Illustrated Reviews: Pharmacology, Sixth Edition.*

This is a condensed pharmacology section to review the most common medications you will use during your rotation. Master these and you will be ahead of the curve.

The amount of medication you give is based on body weight.

The "usual doses" of medications are based on healthy adult patients who are medically stable. Always adjust the medication dose based on the patient, the circumstances, and your anesthetic goals. The following tables list what most would consider to be "reasonable" doses. Most medication doses will be reported as a range. (This drives new anesthesia trainees crazy because it seems that every staff has their own dose that they use in their practice.)

Start at the low end of the range and escalate from there. You can always give more; it is more difficult to "take it back" after it is given to the patient.

Five things to check before giving the medications:
1. Patient medication allergies
   - You don't want to get this one wrong.
   - This can be easily overlooked when you get in a hurry.
2. Patient weight
   - This becomes more important with pediatric anesthesia.
3. Name of the medication
   - Don't go by the look of the vial. Depending on the manufacturer, medications can have similar looking vials, which is the source of most common mistakes.
4. Check the concentration of the medication (mg/ml or mcg/ml)
   - Some medications come in different concentrations.
   - Other medications need to be diluted prior to their administration.
5. Calculate the dose and draw up the proper amount.
   - Use the properly sized syringe.
   - When prepping emergency drugs, only draw up the amount of drug for one unit bolus. This is usually done more often in pediatric anesthesiology.

IV Fluids and Blood

There are three types of IV fluids that you will encounter in the operating room:

1. Crystalloid
2. Colloid
3. Blood products
   - Blood products are colloids as well, but we think of them differently.

Crystalloid Fluids

These are routinely used for patients coming to the OR. The three most common are

- lactated ringers (LR),
- normal saline (NS), and
- plasma-lyte (PL).

Colloid Fluids

These are IV fluids that help pull fluids into the intravascular space. These are used more often when the patients need more volume in their cardiovascular system. The most common are

- Albumin
- Hetastarch

Blood Products

As their name implies, these are products that are given to replace blood loss and the vital blood components that help with coagulation. When you give blood products, typically you need to give them with an IV that is primed with NS or PL. LR is usually not used with blood because it contains calcium and has the potential to cause the blood to clot while in the IV tubing. Blood products you will encounter are

- Packed red blood cells (PRBC)
    - Need to be kept in a cooler until you use them. Because of this, we use a "hot line" (fluid warmer) to administer the blood to warm it up before it is transfused into the patient.
    - Needs to be given through a blood tubing set that has a filter to remove clots and aggregates that have formed.
    - PRBCs can be given with an IV tubing pump.
- Platelets (PLT)
    - Stored at room temperature.
    - Need to be given with a filter set by gravity (IV pumps will destroy the platelets).
- Clotting factors
    - Fresh frozen plasma (FFP)
    - This is the part of the blood that contains the clotting factors needed to form blood clots.
- Cryoprecipitate (Cryo)
    - Contains fibrinogen that is needed to help with clotting as well.

Fluid Replacement

As with medications, IV fluids are given according to the patient's weight in kg.

- The 4-2-1 rule is used to calculate maintenance fluid that the patient should have each hour.
    - 4 ml/kg for the first 10 kg
    - 2 ml/kg for the next 10 kg
    - 1 ml/kg for each kg thereafter
- For example:
    - A 70 kg patient should have "maintenance fluid" of 110 ml/hr.
        - (4 ml x 10 kg) + (2 ml x 10 kg) + (1 ml x 50 kg) = 110 ml/hr.
- A shortcut for patients greater than 20 kg: Add 40 ml to their weight (in kg) to get the maintenance fluid requirement.

When a patient has been without anything to drink, we calculate the amount of maintenance fluid that he or she should received — we call this the patient's fluid deficit.

To calculate the fluid deficit (the amount of fluid the patient is "behind"), we multiply the patient's maintenance requirement by the number of hours he or she has been without fluid. Once the patient has been without fluids for 8 hours, we only calculate the deficit up to 8 hours. This is because most people will concentrate their urine and will not have more than 8 hours' worth of fluid deficit.

For our 70 kg patient above, after a full night's sleep, his fluid deficit would be 880ml because his maintenance fluid rate is 110 ml/hr, and he was without that for more than 8 hours.

Replacing the Deficit:
We replace the fluid deficit during the surgery at the following rate:

- Half given over the first hour
- 1/4 given over the next hour
- 1/4 given over the next hour

We also give the patient his or her regular maintenance fluids during the case as well.   Patients will also lose more body fluids during surgery, depending on the size of the anesthesia case.

- Superficial surgery: 2 ml/kg/hr
- More invasive surgery: 4 ml/kg/hr
- Open bowel surgery: 6 ml/kg/hr

Blood Loss Replacement:
As blood loss is calculated, we replace the blood loss with either crystalloid/colloid or blood at the following ratios:

- 3 ml of crystalloid for each 1 ml of blood loss
- 1 ml of colloid for each 1 ml of blood loss
- 1 ml of PRBC for each 1 ml of blood loss

8. Benzodiazepines and Reversal

Benzodiazepine
Midazolam (Versed)

- A short-acting benzodiazepine commonly used in anesthesia.
- Used in the perioperative period for
  - anxiolysis (prior to surgery)
  - anterograde amnesia (when you need to transport between the OR and the ICU)

Table 2 Benzodiazepines		
Medication	Typical Adult Dose	Pediatric Dose
midazolam (versed)	2 mg IV	0.5 mg/kg PO or 0.1 mg/kg IV (typically up to 2 mg)

Benzodiazepine Reversal
Flumazenil

- Used for reversing the sedative and respiratory depression of a benzodiazepine overdose.
- Use with caution because it can cause seizures in patients from rapid benzodiazepine withdrawal.

Adult dose for reversal of conscious sedation:

- 0.2 mg over 15 seconds
- repeat 0.1 mg q 1 minute to a total of 1 mg

9. Induction Medications

- Used for sedation or induction of general anesthesia.

Propofol (Diprovan)

Drug Class:

- Sterically hindered phenols

Use:

- Very common induction agent
- Also can be used as a sole anesthetic or adjunct anesthetic as an infusion

Advantages:

- Propofol is a reliable induction agent that can also be used to deepen the anesthetic during the case with smaller doses.
- It also has antinausea properties when given as a bolus or an infusion.

Disadvantages:

- It can cause a decrease in blood pressure by reducing systemic vascular resistance and cardiac contractility.
- The patient's blood pressure can decrease dramatically, especially in hypovolemic or dehydrated patients.
- Can cause pain with injection, especially if administered through a poorly working IV
  - The smaller the IV catheter, the more painful the injection.
  - We tend to give lidocaine just prior to the propofol injection to lessen the discomfort, but this does not always work.

- Pushing propofol slowly can also lessen the pain.

Typical Adult Dose:

- 2 mg/kg IV
- 150–200 mg IV push for induction as a standard adult dose
- 1 mg/kg to deepen the anesthesia during the case
- Can be given as an infusion: 100–300 mcg/kg/min.

Etomidate

Drug Class:

- Imidazole derivative

Use:

- It is used as an induction agent for hemodynamically unstable patients.

Advantages:

- Considered more hemodynamically stable than propofol
- Does not reduce systemic vascular resistance like propofol does

Disadvantages:

- Causes adrenal suppression with just one dose
- Cannot be used as an infusion
- Being used less commonly in septic patients because it leads to worse outcomes due to adrenal suppression
- It can also cause myoclonus, pain on injection, and postoperative nausea and vomiting.

Typical Adult Dose:
- 0.2 mg/kg IV
- 14 mg IV push for induction as a standard adult dose
- Rarely used to deepen anesthesia

Ketamine

Drug Class:
- Phyencyclidine (PCP) derivative

Use:
- Can be used as a sole induction agent to induce anesthesia.
- Can also be used as an adjunct to provide analgesia.
- Causes a dissociative anesthesia
  - This is when patients look as if they are awake, but they are not conscious of what is happening around them.

Advantages:
- Can be used when patients are not stable.
- Ketamine can also be given intramuscularly (IM) when an IV cannot be obtained.
- Unlike the other induction medications, ketamine also provides profound analgesia.
- Causes bronchodilation.

Disadvantages:
- May increase intracranial pressure (controversial)
- Associated with emergence delirium and hallucinations.

- We typically give midazolam to help counteract this.
- Ketamine also acts as a sialogogue and increases secretions.
  - We typically give glycopyrrolate or atropine to counteract this.

Typical Adult Ketamine Dose:

- 2 mg/kg IV as an induction dose
- 4 mg/kg IM as an indication dose

May need to also give

- Midazolam (to counteract hallucinations)
- Glycopyrrolate or atropine (to counteract copious oral secretions)

Table 3 Induction Agents		
Medication	Induction Dose	Notes
propofol (10mg/ml)	2 mg/kg	Can cause pain on injection / hypotension is common
etomidate (2mg/ml)	0.2 mg/kg	Maintains hemodynamics / causes adrenal suppression
ketamine (100mg/ml)	2 mg/kg	Increases HR and BP / provides analgesia

10. Pain Medications and Reversals

Opioids

Fentanyl

- Used during induction and throughout surgery to control pain.
- Quick onset and short duration of action make this a good medication to use when surgical conditions are changing.
- *Caution*: Can cause respiratory depression and a rigid chest syndrome that can interfere with breathing.
- Time to peak effect: 5 min. (IV)
- Duration: 45 min.

Typical Adult Dose:

- 0.5–1 mcg/kg on induction
- 1 mcg/kg during surgery for pain

Morphine

- Typically used toward the end of surgery
- Causes less respiratory depression than fentanyl
- Lasts longer than fentanyl
- *Caution*: Can cause a histamine release in some patients that leads to itching and hives.
- Time to peak effect: 20 min. (IV)
- Duration: 4 hours

Typical Adult Morphine Dose:

- 2 mg / dose — titrated to respiratory rate
- A respiratory rate of "8 is great, 10 I'll take." This reminds us that a spontaneous respiratory rate of 8–10 usually indicates adequate analgesia.

Hydromorphone (Dilaudid)

- It is a synthetic derivative of morphine.
- Causes less histamine release than morphine.
- *Caution*: More potent than morphine; the patient will require a lower dose than morphine.
- Time to peak effect: 20 min. (IV)
- Duration: 4–5 hours

Typical Adult Dose:

- 0.01 mg/kg/dose
- 0.2 mg / dose — titrated to respiratory rate

Meperidine

- Most commonly used to combat postoperative rigors (shivering related to anesthesia) in the PACU
- Time to peak effect: 15 min.
- Duration: 2 hours

Typical Adult Dose:

- 12.5 mg — may be repeated once

Table 4 Common Opioids					
Medication	Est. Potency	Typical Adult Dose	Pediatric Dose (pain)	Peak Affect	Duration
fentanyl	100	25–50 mcg	0.5–1 mcg/kg/dose	5 min.	45 min.
morphine	1	2–4 mg	0.05–0.1 mg/kg/dose	20 min.	4 hrs.
hydromorphone	10	0.2 mg	0.01 mg/kg/dose	20 min.	5 hrs.
meperidine	0.1	12.5 mg	1–2 mg/kg	15 min.	2 hrs.

Opioid Reversal

Naloxone

- Used for reversing the sedative and respiratory depression of a relative opioid overdose.
- If it is used to reverse a long-acting opioid, then it may "wear off" before the opioid effects do and may require re-dosing.
- *Caution*: Can cause flash pulmonary edema.
- Onset: 2 min.
- Duration: 30 min.

Typical Adult Nalozone Dose:

- 0.04 mg IV

Table 5 Opioid Reversal			
Medication	Adult Dose	Onset	Duration
naloxone	0.04 mg IV	1–2 min.	30 min.

Non-Opioid Pain Medication

Acetaminophen

- Can be given either IV or PO
- *Caution*: Make sure the patient is not on other acetaminophen-containing medications before you give acetaminophen.

Typical Adult Dose: (Not to exceed 4 grams in a 24 hr. period)

- 15 mg/kg not to exceed 1 gram IV q 6 hours
- 650 mg PO q 6 hours

Ibuprofen

- NSAID
- Usually given PO in the United States
- *Caution*: Be careful not to give it to a patient who is also taking ketorolac because taking both ibuprofen and ketorolac at the same time can cause kidney problems.

Typical Adult Ibuprofen Dose:

- 600 mg PO

Ketorolac

- NSAID
- Can be given IV or IM
- *Caution*: Be careful not to give it to a patient who is also taking ibuprofen.
- Make sure the patient is well hydrated because it can cause decreased renal blood flow.

Typical Adult Dose:

- IM/IV 30 mg then 15–30 mg q 6 hours

Table 6 Non-Opioid Pain Medications			
Medication	Adult PO Dose	Adult IV Dose	Comments
acetaminophen	650 mg q 6 hrs.	1 gram q hr.	Use caution with other medications that contain acetaminophen
ilbuprofen	600 mg q 6 hrs.	- - -	Do not give with Ketorolac
ketorolac	- - -	30 mg then 15–30 mg q 6 hrs.	Do not give with Ibuprofen

11. Neuromuscular Blocking Medications and Reversals

- Neuromuscular blockers (NMB) or "muscle relaxants" are utilized to chemically paralyze skeletal muscle at the neuromuscular junction. These drugs chemically relax the skeletal muscles to allow the surgeon to operate or keep the patient from trying to breathe against a ventilator.

- The effects of the NMB are monitored with a twitch monitor that sends an electrical impulse through a nerve. You evaluate the response to a group of four twitches (called a "train of four" or TOF). TOF and the ability to maintain sustained tetany will help you determine how much the NMB is affecting the patient.

- The use of muscle relaxants is the most common cause of anaphylaxis in patients going to the OR.

There are two types of neuromuscular blocking medications:

- Depolarizing, which causes depolarization of the muscle (i.e., uncoordinated movements [fasciculations] when the medication is given)

- Non-depolarizing, which does not cause depolarization of the muscle (i.e., no perceivable movement when the medication is given).

Depolarizing Medications

Succinylcholine (Sux)

Advantages:

- Sux has the most rapid onset and shortest duration of action of all the paralytics.
- Commonly used in rapid sequence inductions (RSI). (See ch. 27 for a discussion on RSI.)

Disadvantages:

- Contraindicated in burn and stroke patients because of related lethal hyperkalemia due to extra-junctional acetylcholine receptors.
- With severe burns and stroke, the muscle cells increase the number of acetylcholine receptors that are located outside the neuromuscular junction. When Sux is given to these patients, it cases a massive release of potassium with the muscle depolarization.
- When the dose is pushed up to 2 mg/kg, your patients can have myalgia after waking up or the day after anesthesia.
- Sux is also one of the triggers of malignant hyperthermia (See ch. 31, "Malignant Hyperthermia.")

Typical Adult Dose:

- 1–2 mg/kg
- 180 mg IV push

Non-Depolarizing Medications:

Vecuronium (Vec)

Advantages:

- Commonly used because it is cheap.
- Has a very reliable duration of action.

Disadvantages:

- Comes as a powder that has to be reconstituted with sterile water.

Typical Adult Dose:

- 0.1 mg/kg
- 15 mg IV push as a standard adult dose

Rocuronium (Roc)

Advantages:

- Commonly used because it is quick to draw up (already in solution).
- Best alternative when Sux is contraindicated to intubate with a modified RSI because of its fast onset.

Disadvantages:

- Tends to be more expensive than Sux and Vec.
- It has been reported that some patients have muscles weakness leading to respiratory depression after surgery.

Typical Adult Dose:

- 0.6 mg/kg
- 50 mg IV push as a standard adult dose
- When used for a modified RSI, 1.2 mg/kg

Cisatracurium (Cis)

Advantages:

- Used with patients who have renal disease or failure because it does not rely on the liver or kidney for metabolism/elimination.

Disadvantages:

- If used after Roc (as with a modified RSI), then the elimination of Cis is not as predictable.

Typical Adult Dose:

- 0.2 mg/kg
- 14 mg IV push as a standard adult dose

Table 7 Muscle Relaxants				
Medication	Typical Adult Dose	Intubating Dose	Onset	Duration
succinylcholine	180 mg	1–2 mg/kg	1 min.	5–10 min.
vecuronium	15 mg	0.1–0.2 mg/kg	3–5 min.	20–35 min.
rocuronium	50 mg	0.6 mg/kg	1–2 min.	20–35 min.
cisatracurium	14 mg	0.2 mg/kg	1–2 min.	60 min.

Neuromuscular Reversal Agents

Neuromuscular reversal agents are given to patients who received a non-depolarizing neuromuscular blocker after the return of at least one twitch with the twitch monitor.

Neostigmine

Neostigmine is an anticholinesterase medication that increases the amount of acetylcholine throughout the body.

Do not confuse "Neo," the slang term for neosynephrine, for neostigmine (See ch. 13).

Neostigmine works by increasing the amount of acetylcholine at the neuromuscular junction, which causes reversal of the neuromuscular blockade.

Side effects of neostigmine include bradycardia and SLUDGE (salivation, lacrimation, urination, defecation, GI upset, and emesis).

Typical Adult Dose:

- 0.07 mg/kg up to 5 mg
- The dose may be decreased depending on the measure of TOF. Giving too much reversal can cause weakness as well. I recommend discussing the dose with your staff or preceptor.

Glycopyrrolate

- Given along with the neostigmine to offset its side effects of bradycardia and SLUDGE symptoms.
- Calculate the dose of neostigmine, and then use the same volume of glycopyrrolate for a quick calculation.

Typical Adult Dose:

- 0.2 mg/kg for every 1 mg neostigmine given, up to 1 mg total glycopyrrolate

For example:

You calculate that the patient should receive 4 mg of neostigmine (which is 4 ml), and then you would use 4 ml of glycopyrrolate (which is 0.8 mg with a concentration of 0.2 mg/ml).

Table 8 Relaxant Reversal			
Medication	Dose	Max dose	Max Volume
neostigmine	0.05–0.07 mg/kg	5 mg	5 ml
glycopyrrolate	0.2 mg for every 1 mg of neostigmine given	1 mg	5 ml

12. Autonomic Nervous System Medications

"Not too high, not too low. Not too fast, not too slow."
> — A typical cardiologist's "cardiac recommendations."

Basic Cardiovascular Physiology
Thus, there are four factors that affect blood pressure (BP):

1. heart rate (HR)
2. preload
3. contractility
4. afterload

Heart rate (HR) and blood pressure (BP) are related to the following formulas:

$$BP = CO \times SVR$$

$$BP = (HR \times SV) \times SVR$$

$$BP = (HR \times (LVEDV\text{-}LVESV)) \times SVR \text{ or } BP = (HR \times (preload \text{ - } contractility)) \times afterload,$$

where
CO = cardiac output
SVR = systemic vascular resistance
SV = stroke volume
HR = heart rate
LVEDV = left ventricular end-diastolic volume
LVESV = left ventricular end-systolic volume

Once you understand this formula, you can see how changing one variable can affect the rest of the parameters. For example, if you give phenylephrine (an alpha 1 agonist that ↑ SVR) to a patient with hypotension (↓ BP) and tachycardia (↑ HR), then the BP should increase (due to ↑ SVR), which will lead to a reflexive decrease in HR because the HR is no longer trying to maintain the BP.

Vasoactive Drugs Can be Dangerous

Vasoactive medications typically increase or decrease HR, BP, and SVR; these are the medications we use to keep the HR and BP within 20% of the preoperative values.

These medications can be some of our most dangerous medications because they typically come very concentrated. Most of the time, you have to dilute these drugs at least once before giving them! Not diluting these drugs can lead to *killing someone*.

Make sure you do this the right way and LABEL THE CONCENTRATION on the syringe.

Diluting Medications

Single Dilution

- Used most often for ephedrine.
    1. Start with the concentrated vial of medication.
    2. Draw up 1 ml of the concentrated medication and add 9 ml of normal saline (NS) to it.
    3. The new concentration will now be 1/10 of the original concentration with a total volume of 10 ml.

Single dilution example:

1. Start with 50 mg/ml of ephedrine in a 1 ml vial.
2. Draw up the 1 ml of ephedrine and add 9 ml of NS to it.
3. The 50 mg is now in 10 ml of solution, so the new concentration is now 5 mg/ml.

Double Dilution

- Used most often for phenylephrine and epinephrine.

Method One (Two-Syringe Method)

1. Start with the ultra-concentrated vial of medication.
4. Draw up 1 ml of the concentrated medication and add 9 ml of NS to it.
5. The new concentration will now be 1/10 of the original, with a total volume of 10 ml.
6. Draw up 1 ml of the new concentration (1/10) and add 9 ml of NS to it.
7. The new concentration will now be 1/100 of the original, with a total volume of 10 ml.

Double dilution example:

1. Start with the ultra-concentrated medication (10 mg/ml of Neosynephrine).
2. Draw up 1 ml of the 10 mg/ml and add 9 ml of NS to it.
3. Your new super concentrated medication is now 1 mg/ml, <u>which is still too high</u>.
4. Take 1 ml of that solution of the new super concentration (1 mg/ml) and put it into another 9 ml of NS.
5. The new concentration will be 0.1 mg/ml, or more commonly called 100 mcg/ml.

Method Two (100 ml bag of NS)

This is a great method for getting a double dilution very quickly and making sure syringe swaps don't happen.

1. Take 1 ml of NS out of a 100 ml bag of NS.
2. Put in the 1 ml of your ultra-concentrated drug (10 mg/ml of phenylephrine).
3. **Bam:** 100 ml of double diluted medication − 100 mcg/ml.

The Key to Proper Dilutions:

1. Know your starting concentration.
2. For each 1 ml of the starting concentration put into 9 ml of NS, move the decimal one place to the left.

Label everything with the concentration you know to be correct. If you get confused or don't remember, then trash it and start over. <u>Do only one dilution at a time</u>. This is not the time to multitask.

Autonomic Nervous System Receptors

Knowing what each type of autonomic receptor does will help you to understand how each drug you use affects your patients. The table below is a quick review of the receptors you have probably learned about in your past basic physiology courses.

Table 9 Adrenoceptors for Pressors			
Receptor	Location	Agonist Action	Antagonist Action
alpha - 1	Peripheral blood vessels	↑ SVR	-
alpha - 2	End of nerve	Inhibits norepi release	-
	centrally in the brain		
beta - 1	Heart	↑HR and ↑contractility	↓HR and ↓contractility
beta - 2	Lungs	Broncho-dilation	Broncho-constriction
	vascular smooth muscle	vaso-dilation	-

13. Vasoactive Medications ("Pressors")

Catecholamine

Epinephrine (Epi)

- Old school name = adrenaline
- This is a "big gun" — start with lower doses and titrate to effect
- Direct acting catecholamine (alpha1, beta1, and beta2)
- Increases HR and SVR, which increase BP

Dilution to get to 0.01 mg/ml = 10 mcg/ml

A 1 mg/ml Epi (small ampule) will require a double dilution. A 0.1 mg/ml Epi (Bristoject™) will require a single dilution. Either way should get you to a concentration of 0.01 mg/ml = 10 mcg/ml.

Typical Adult Dose:

- 10 mcg IV push
- These are not "code doses." These are small titrations to get an effect.

Sympathomimetics

Ephedrine
- Don't confuse with epinephrine
- Used routinely in adult anesthesia
- Indirect acting sympathomimetic (alpha1 and beta1)
    - Stimulates the release of catecholamine stores in the patient.
- Increases HR and SVR, which increase BP

Will need dilution to get to 5 mg/ml

Typically comes as 50 mg/ml — single dilution to 5 mg/ml

Typical Adult Dose:
- 5 mg IV push

Phenylephrine (Neo)
Called "Neo" because the trade name is Neosynephrine™

- Used routinely in adult anesthesia
- Direct acting agent (alpha1 agonist)
- Increases SVR, which increases BP
- It can cause a reflexive decrease in HR when the BP increases.
    - This might be the first change in vital signs you see.
- Use with caution if HR is low because it may cause a further reduction in HR.

Phenylephrine needs dilution to get to 0.1 mg/ml = 100 mcg/ml unless it comes in a prefilled syringe:

Typically comes as 10 mg/ml and requires a **double dilution** to get to 0.1 mg/ml (100 mcg/ml).

Adult Starting Dose:
- 50 to 100 mcg IV push

Table 10 Vasoactive Drugs			
Medication	Dilution	Concentration	Adult Starting Dose
epinephrine	single or double	10 mcg/ml	10 mcg
ephedrine	single	5 mg/ml	5 mg
phenylephrine	double	100 mcg/ml	50–100 mcg

14. Antihypertensives

These are used to lower HR and BP.

Esmolol

- Pure beta blocker (beta1 antagonist)
- Fast acting and has a short duration of action

Adult Starting Dose:

- 10 mg IV push q 3 min. as needed

Labetalol

- Alpha and beta blocker
- Fast acting and has a long duration

Adult Starting Dose:

- 5 mg IV push q 5 min. as needed

Metoprolol

- Beta 1 selective
- Longer acting than esmolol

Adult Starting Dose:

- 2.5 mg IV push q 2 min. as needed

Table 11 Antihypertensives			
Medication	Concentration	Adult Starting Dose	Elimination Half Life
esmolol	10 mg/ml	10 mg	10 min.
labetalol	5 mg/ml	5 mg	5.5 hrs.
metoprolol	1 mg /ml	2.5 mg	3.5 hrs.

15. Common Antibiotics

Preoperative antibiotics are commonly ordered by surgeons but administered by the anesthesia team. In adult anesthesia or those patients who have an IV prior to induction, the antibiotic should be in the patient 30 minutes prior to surgery incision to decrease postoperative skin infections. In pediatric patients, where the IV is typically started after induction, then the antibiotic is given as soon as possible after the IV is started.

Some anesthesiologists give a small "test dose" before giving the total dose to make sure patients don't have an allergic reaction. The most common spot to notice histamine release is in mast cells on the anterior chest. If there was a histamine release, then you would expect to see redness and possibly urticaria develop.

Table 12 Common Antibiotics		
Antibiotics	Adult Dose	Pediatric Dose
ampicillin	1–2 grams IV	25 mg/Kg
cefazolin (ancef)	1–2 grams IV	25 mg/Kg
clindamycin	600 mg	10 mg/Kg
gentamicin *	120 mg divided q 6 hrs.	1.5 mg/Kg
metronidazole (Flagyl)	500 mg IV q 8 hrs.	30 mg/kg/day
vancomycin **	1 gram IV	10 mg/kg
* give slowly to avoid ringing in the ears and ototoxicity		
** give slowly to avoid "red man" syndrome due to histamine release		

16. Common Local Anesthetics

These medications block the transmission of neurons by blocking sodium channels. Each local anesthetic has a slightly different onset, risk profile, and duration of action. The most important thing to remember with local anesthetics is that although they are used very often and safely, they each have a toxic dose. Local toxicity can manifest as either central nervous system toxicity or cardiovascular system toxicity.

Table 13 Common Local Anesthetics			
Local Anesthesia	Max Dose Plain	Max Dose with Epi	Onset
bupivacaine	2.5 mg/kg	3 mg/kg	5–15 min.
lidocaine	4.5 mg/kg	7 mg/kg	5–15 min.
ropivacaine	2.5 mg/kg	2.5 mg/kg	10–20 min.

17. Postoperative Nausea and Vomiting (PONV)

One of the most frustrating side effects of anesthesia, for both you and the patient, is postoperative nausea and vomiting (PONV). There are several things you can do to decrease the chances of PONV. This is especially important for high-risk patients. You can determine a high-risk patient by the number of risk factors your patient has. For each risk factor, there is an increase in the chances of PONV; up to 80% in some studies! There are several risk factors in adults that can predict risk of PONV:

Patient Factors
1. Female gender
2. Nonsmoker
3. History of PONV
4. History of motion sickness
5. < 50 y/o

Anesthesia/Surgery Factors
1. Use of volatile anesthesia
2. Use of N2O
3. Duration of anesthesia
4. Type of surgery
5. Use of opioids intraoperatively
6. Postoperative use of opioids

Strategies you can use to reduce the risk of PONV:
1. Use more regional anesthesia (See ch. 30) instead of general anesthesia
2. Use propofol for induction and continue it as an infusion during the case
3. Avoid volatile anesthesia
4. Avoid N2O

5. Minimize intraoperative and postoperative opioids
6. Keep the patient appropriately hydrated
7. Use medications for prevention and rescue of PONV (see below)

PONV Medications Commonly Used
Dexamethasone
Dexamethasone is a steroid that is typically given at induction of anesthesia to prevent PONV. Make sure you give it *after* the patient is asleep. Patients can have an intense burning in apocrine glands on IV push. (Their armpits and genitals burn like crazy as a side effect.)
Typical Adult Dose:
- 4 mg IV

Ondansetron
A 5-HT3 receptor antagonist. It is better at preventing vomiting than preventing nausea.
Typical Adult Dose:
- 4 mg IV or 8 mg PO as an oral dissolving tablet (ODT)

My PONV Recipe for the High-Risk Patient:
Pre-Op
- midazolam
  - To help prevent recall

Intra-Op
- No N2O
- Dexamethasone — 0.15 mg/kg up to 4 mg IV on induction
- Propofol infusion — 100 mcg/kg/min. during the case as a background infusion

- Dexmedetomidine 0.5 – 1 mcg/kg as a load over 10 minutes
  - Reduces the amount of opioid you need to give.
- Acetaminophen IV 15 mg/kg if < 50 kg or 1 gram if > 50 kg
  - Reduces the amount of opioid you need to give.
- Sevoflurane in Air/O2
  - To help prevent recall
- 10–20 ml/kg of LR if there is no contraindication
- Ondansetron 0.15 mg/kg up to 8 mg IV at the end

Post-Op

- Sips of clear liquids in PACU slowly
- Inform the person driving the patient home to be careful when driving to minimize motion sickness as much as possible.

Table 14 PONV Medications – Adult Doses		
Medication	Dose	When to Give
dexamethasone	4 mg IV	At induction
ondansetron	4 mg IV or 8 mg ODT	At end of surgery or as a rescue in the PACU

18. Preoperative Anesthesia H&P

Getting Ready for Surgery

The preoperative period is one of the most underappreciated parts of patient care for students. Many times, anesthesia students want to "get to the fun stuff" and get on with the induction of anesthesia.

Part of our job as the anesthesia team is to anticipate problems so we can avoid them. When you avoid problems, you don't have to fix them. Think of it as going around a hole instead of going into a hole and having to be pulled out.

A good preoperative evaluation makes sure the patient is physically and emotionally ready for surgery and there are no unaddressed health issues. In emergency surgery, you don't have time to optimize the patient. For elective or semi-elective surgery, you will have time to medically optimize the patient before getting to the OR.

The other part of getting ready for surgery is to develop an anesthetic plan based on the needs of the patient and the needs of the surgery. Although your anesthetic plan may change in the middle of surgery, you must always have a plan in place before induction. Many times you will have a plan, plus several backup plans, in place before your induction.

The anesthesia history and physical (H&P) is designed to find specific problems that are of interest to the anesthesia team. It is also the time to build a rapport with the patient and their family and gain their confidence.

The Anesthesia History

The following should be considered in the anesthesia H&P.

- Airway
- Obstructive sleep apnea (OSA)
    - Risk factors include body mass index (BMI) > 30, neck circumference > 40 cm, hypertension (HTN), snoring, observed apnea, daytime somnolence, male gender, and nocturia.
- **STOP-Bang acronym** (risk factors are additive)
    - Snoring (loud snoring)
    - Tired (daytime sleepiness)
    - Observed (observed stopped breathing during sleep)
    - Pressure (high blood pressure)
    - BMI (greater than 35)
    - Age (greater than 50)
    - Neck circumference (greater than 40 cm)
- Heart
    - Coronary artery disease (CAD)
    - Coronary artery bypass graph (CABG)
    - Coronary stent placement
    - Murmur
    - HTN
    - Exercise tolerance
    - Taking any aspirin or antiplatelet drugs
- Lungs

- Chronic obstructive pulmonary disease (COPD)
- Asthma
- Liver problems
- Kidney problems
  - Acute renal issues
  - Chronic kidney disease (CKD)
  - Renal failure
- Endocrine
- Diabetes (DM)
  - On insulin or oral medications?
  - Does the patient have an insulin pump?
- Oral steroid use
- Social
  - Smoker
  - Alcohol use/abuse
  - Street drugs
- Current Medications
  - What current medications is the patient taking at home?
  - Why is he or she taking them?
- Allergies
  - Medication allergies
  - Food allergies (esp. egg and soy; many preparations of propofol contain egg lecithin and/or soy)
  - Latex allergies?
- Surgical/anesthesia history
  - Family problems with anesthesia?

- Especially a family history of malignant hyperthermia (see chapter 32)
- Patient problems with past anesthesia?
    - PONV?
- NPO status (see chart below)
    - Last meal (when and what they last ate)
    - Last fluid intake (when and what they last drank)

I make it a habit to ask, "Are there any other health problems that we have not talked about?" Once in a while this question will catch something that the patient forgot to tell you.

Anesthesia Physical Exam

Airway Exam (see chapter 19, "Airway Exam and Assessment")

- Heart
    - Do they have a regular rate and rhythm?
    - Any murmurs?
    - Do the heart tones and pulse match up?
- Lungs
    - Good air movement?
    - Any decreased air movement?
    - Any wheezes or rales?
- Peripheral pulses
    - Especially the radial arteries (for starting arterial lines)
    - Are they right- or left-hand dominant (for placement of A-line in the nondominant hand)

- Easily identifiable peripheral veins (for starting IVs)
  - Particularly the upper extremities

Preoperative Labs / Studies

For most healthy patients undergoing low risk procedures, no labs are needed.

The need for preoperative tests / labs is based on

1. the patient's current health, and
2. the surgery that will be performed.

The one exception to this rule is the pregnancy test.

Pregnancy Test

Every female of childbearing age should have a urine pregnancy test. If they can't provide a urine sample, then you should obtain a human chorionic gonadotropin (hCG) blood test. If your patient is pregnant, then you need to determine the risk of proceeding; the urgency of the surgery and the postconceptional age of the fetus must be determined. If you need to proceed, then avoid the following:

1. midazolam (and other benzodiazepines) because of the risk for fetal cleft lip and palate
2. N2O because it inhibits methionine synthase and affects DNA synthesis. The concern is that neurological development could be affected and lead to birth defects.

If the patient is far enough along in her pregnancy to deliver a viable baby, then you also need to do intraoperative fetal monitoring and have facilities available to emergently delivery the baby.

ASA Physical Status

Once your H&P is complete, you can assign the patient an American Society of Anesthesiologists (ASA) physical status.

ASA I - "A normal healthy patient"

ASA II - "A patient with mild systemic disease"

ASA III - "A patient with severe systemic disease"

ASA IV - "A patient with severe systemic disease that is a constant threat to life"

ASA V - "A moribund patient who is not expected to survive without the operation"

ASA VI - "A declared brain-dead patient whose organs are being removed for donor purposes"

E - A modifier added to the ASA status to describe a case that is not scheduled as an elective case.

NPO Guidelines

Nil per os (NPO) — nothing per mouth — this is the time from their last oral intake until they have an expected empty stomach. It is imperative that patients have an empty stomach because if there's food/liquid in their stomach, it could be aspirated into the lungs. Aspiration can cause pneumonia or, worse, a fatal event. This is why we have patients NPO for surgery.

If the surgery is an emergency and there is not sufficient time to wait for the appropriate NPO time, then we use a procedure called a rapid sequence induction (RSI) to place in an endotracheal tube (ETT) to protect the lungs (see chapter 27, "RSI").

Table 15 NPO Times	
Clear liquids (including black coffee and pulp-free clear juice)	2 hrs.
Breast milk (with nothing mixed into it)	4 hrs.
Light meal (dry toast, bread, crackers, cow's milk)	6 hrs.
Heavy meal (greasy foods, large meal)	8 hrs.
*Patients with decreased gastric emptying may need longer times.	
**Trauma patients (and those patients in pain) have decreased gastric motility and make NPO less relevant. These patients are treated as if they have a full stomach.	

19. Airway Exam and Assessment

The airway exam is done in an effort to predict when you might encounter a difficult mask ventilation and/or intubation. It should be done on every patient undergoing anesthesia or an intubation procedure. The airway exam should be done in the seated position, whenever possible. This exam has only been validated in adults, but parts of it can be used to evaluate pediatric patients as well.

There are four basic parts to the airway exam:

1. Neck extension and flexion
   - Have the patient flex and extend his or her head.
      - Limited movement may indicate difficulty with intubation.

2. Thyromental distance
   - Assess how many finger breadths from the patient's thyroid notch to the end of his or her chin.
      - A shorter thyromental distance can indicate a more difficult intubation.

3. Mouth opening
   - Any limitations to opening their mouth?

4. Mallampati class
   - This describes what the inside of the mouth looks like. The higher the Mallampati class, the higher the probability of a difficult intubation.

When the patient opens his or her mouth while in the seated position, you can see the following:

- Class I - soft palate, fauces, uvula, and tonsillar pillars
- Class II - soft palate, fauces, and uvula
- Class III - soft palate and base of uvula
- Class IV - only the hard palate is visible

Any one indicator does not, by itself, predict a potentially difficult airway. The four indicators should be taken together to predict possible issues with the patient's airway. This is important when the patient has had surgery or radiation to the head or neck.

Pediatric Airway Exam

The airway exam, particularly the Mallampati class, has not been validated in infants and children. Mostly, what you will be able to obtain in pediatric patients is

- thyromental distance,
- maybe neck extension, and
- maybe mouth opening.

20. Presenting Your Patient to Your Staff or Preceptor

You will need to learn how to be a good, if not great, verbal communicator when working in the field of anesthesia. And part of this begins with your interactions with your staff/preceptor.

There are times during your rotation that you will complete an anesthesia H&P, come up with an anesthetic plan, and present the information to your staff/preceptor who is overseeing you. You are trying to paint a picture of how healthy (or unhealthy) the patient is, what kind of procedure he or she will be having, and your anesthetic plan.

One way to present your patient is to start with a summary sentence (see below) and then proceed in a SOAP format:

> S - Subjective (what you are told — the patient's history)
>
> O - Objective (what you find on physical exam)
> > • Start with the airway exam, and then give the physical exam.
>
> A - Assessment (this is where you put together the H&P into a total picture of the patient)
>
> P - Plan (your anesthetic plan)

An alternative way of presenting is by systems. Start with the summary sentence (see below), and then go through each organ system (airway, cardiac, pulmonary, gastrointestinal, endocrine, neuro, other), detailing H&P exam findings. Then end with your anesthetic plan.

An example of a summary sentence: "This is a _____ -year-old (y/o) _____ (male or female) with/without a significant past medical history of _____ here for a _____ surgery."

The better you present the patient, the more confidence you will instill in your staff or preceptor and the better your chances will be to do more procedures and more direct patient care.

When you first start, you may not have much of an anesthetic plan because you don't know what to do. This is OK. You can simply state that you plan on a regional anesthetic or a general anesthetic and have the preceptor or staff guide you in what to do. As you advance through your training, you will gain more experience and confidence and will be able to deliver your patient presentation along with your plan more efficiently.

21. Anesthesia Machine and Monitors

This chapter is best read after a strong cup of coffee. It will make much more sense to you after you have spent time in the OR working with the anesthesia machine.

The anesthesia machine is perhaps one of the most intimidating pieces of equipment we use. Each machine, although a little different, will have the same basic parts. A machine check should be completed prior to giving an anesthetic (see ch. 22, "Setting Up Your Room").

Basically, each machine has four parts:

1. Medical gases — most commonly air, N2O, and O2

   The flow of the gasses go as follows: pipeline (or tanks) -> flow meters -> vaporizers -> breathing apparatus -> patient

   • If you want a more rapid change in your anesthesia vapors, increase the flows of the gas.

   • The higher the total gas flow, the faster the percentage change in vapor.

2. Vaporizers — Isoflurane, Sevoflorane, Desflurane

   • Each vaporizer is anesthesia vapor specific and will turn the liquid anesthetic into a vapor.

   • Don't fill a vaporizer with the wrong vapor because that will mix the vapor drugs and cause it not to work properly.

- Desflurane vaporizer needs power to work because Des needs to be warmed up to reach a vapor state.

3. Breathing apparatus—anesthesia circuit, "hand bag," ventilator

    The gas flows through the vaporizer; the mixture then flows to your patient. Your patient inhales, and then exhales a mixture of some of the vapor, gas, and CO_2. This mixture flows from the patient, back to the anesthesia machine, through a CO_2 absorbent, and is mixed with fresh gas/vapor that is being added to the system. Much of the gas/vapor mixture is circulated between the patient and the machine. Because fresh gas/vapor is continually being added to the system, the extra gas is removed from the system, via the scavenging system. If you lower the fresh gas flow, then the patient is rebreathing more of the mixture. If you raise the fresh gas flow, then the patient is rebreathing less of the mixture.

    - There are two basic ways to ventilate the patient: manually with the hand bag or with the machine.
    - The hand bag is used to manually ventilate the patient, or to allow him or her to breathe spontaneously (the patient breathes on his or her own).

- The machine can assist the patient or completely breathe for your patient depending on your anesthesia machine.
- Familiarize yourself with how to turn on/off the various machine modes.

4. Monitors

   When you first go in the room, look at the monitor to determine where each vital sign is located on the monitor (every brand of monitor is a little different). The standard ASA monitors are SpO2, HR, ECG, BP, EtCO2, Temperature, and Oxygen Analyzer on the anesthesia machine.

Basic Monitors

- Pulse Oximetry (SpO2)
  - This monitor gives you two important pieces of information:
    - Heart rate
    - The amount of oxygen in the blood
- ECG −3 or 5 lead
  - Records the electrical activity of the heart
  - We typically monitor Lead II. If you're concerned about heart disease, then monitor Lead II along with V5 to capture 95% of electrical activity of the heart.
- Non-Invasive Blood Pressure (BP cuff)
  - This is the BP cuff that inflates/deflates to give you a BP measurement.

- End Tidal CO2 (EtCO2)
    - This is the amount of CO2 being exhaled by the patient.
- Gas Analysis
    - Tells you how much N2O, O2, and anesthesia vapors are going to the patient (inspiratory) and coming from the patient (expiratory).
- Temperature
    - The patient's temperature — usually axillary, nasopharyngeal, or esophageal.
- Muscle Twitch Monitor (Peripheral Nerve Stimulator)
    - Tests skeletal muscle paralytics

Advanced Monitor
- BIS Monitor
    - This monitor is used to try to determine level of consciousness (LOC) in patients.
    - Electroencephalogram (EEG) waves are recorded from the patient and interpreted by the computer and a number is produced that should correlate with level of consciousness.

- BIS scores and relevance:
    - 100 – awake
    - 70–100 – light/moderate sedation
    - 60–70 – deep sedation
    - 40–0 – general anesthesia
    - < 40 – deep hypnotic state
    - 0 – EEG at flat line

Invasive Monitors
- Arterial line (A-line)
    - Provides a measured BP with every heartbeat.
- Central Line
    - This is a centrally placed (placed in a large vein) catheter that can give IV fluids and can also measure central venous pressure (CVP) with the proper monitoring set up.

- Pulmonary artery catheter (Swan or Swan-Ganz catheter)
  - This is a monitor that is placed through an introducer into a large vein, which will enter the heart and go through the right atrium, right ventricle, and end up in the pulmonary artery.
  - With this monitor you can measure the following:
    - CVP
    - Cardiac output
    - Oxygen content of the blood in the central circulation
    - Various pressures within the heart

22. Setting Up Your Room

Use the acronym "MS-MAIDS" so that you make sure you have everything ready for the patient. We use the MS-MAIDS before we start each case. We usually do a full machine check before the first case of the day, and then we do an abbreviated one between cases.

As you set up your work station, try to keep it clean and organized. It will make finding the right medication/equipment at the right time easier. Also, as you prepare your equipment, which come in sterile packaging (ETT and LMA come to mind), open the package but don't lay the equipment out on a non-sterile field. That equipment is sterile for a reason, so please try and keep it that way.

PMS-MAIDS

P - positioning

M - machine check

S - suction

M - monitors

A - airway

I - intravenous equipment

D - drugs

S - special blood, special monitors

- seat—seriously, you don't want to stand the whole time

Positioning:

Do you need any special equipment to position the patient properly, such as a ramp for large patients or a face pillow for prone cases?

Machine Check:

2008 ASA Guidelines for Pre-Anesthesia Checkout Procedures:

1. Verify auxiliary oxygen cylinder and self-inflating manual ventilation device are available and functioning.
2. Verify patient suction is adequate to clear the airway.
3. Turn on anesthesia delivery system and confirm that AC power is available.
4. Verify availability of required monitors and check alarms.
5. Verify that pressure is adequate on the spare oxygen cylinder mounted on the anesthesia machine.
6. Verify that piped gas pressures are ≥ 50 psig.
7. Verify that vaporizers are adequately filled and, if applicable, that the filler ports are tightly closed.
8. Verify that there are no leaks in the gas supply lines between the flow meters and the common gas outlet.
9. Test scavenging system function.
10. Calibrate, or verify calibration of, the oxygen monitor and check the low oxygen alarm.
11. Verify carbon dioxide absorbent is not exhausted.
12. Breathing system pressure and leak testing.

- Part of this is the high pressure check
  - You close the airway pressure limiting (APL) valve, put your thumb over the breathing circuit tube to occlude it, press the O2 flush button until 40 cm H2O pressure is built up. You then watch the airway pressure gauge to see whether the system will maintain the pressure.

13. Verify that gas flows properly through the breathing circuit during both inspiration and exhalation.
14. Document completion of checkout procedures.
15. Confirm ventilator settings and evaluate readiness to deliver anesthesia care.

Also, do you have the proper sized mask and ventilation bag? (I am a pediatric anesthesiologists, what can I say?)

For the abbreviated machine check, we typically do a high pressure check (as described above) and make sure we have plenty of liquid anesthesia gas in the vaporizers. The best way to understand a machine check is to see one.

Suction:

Is it present and working? Although it is checked in the "machine check," it is one of the most overlooked things people forget until they really need it.

Monitors:

Check all your standard monitors. Do you have all the cables for your ECG, BP, pulse, and check to make sure your $EtCO_2$ is present and functioning.

Airway:

Before you start a case, you should have a plan about how you will provide your anesthetic. You may have a primary plan of using an LMA, but you should also be prepared with an endotracheal tube, in case the LMA does not work well. Also, if the patient has a potentially difficult airway, then you might have an LMA available for rescue.

Have your primary airway instruments ready to go and your backup airway supplies easily accessible but kept in the package.

- Laryngoscope
- Handle
    - Properly sized blades
    - Do the blades work with the handle?
- Oral pharyngeal airway (OPA)
- Nasal pharyngeal airway (NPA)
    - Also called nasal trumpets
- Laryngeal mask airway (LMA)
- Endotracheal tubes (ETT)

Intravenous Equipment:

- IV start kit
- IV bag and tubing

Drugs:

- Draw up medications based on your anesthetic plan.
- Hold on to your medication vials so that can always go back and check that you have the correct medications drawn up.
- Label all your syringes and make sure the concentration is easily seen.

- Remember some of your medications
  will be double diluted. Don't get the
  syringes confused (see ch. 23,
  "Common Adult Set Up at Teaching
  Hospitals").

Special Blood/Special Monitors / Seat:

- Advanced monitors
  - If available:
    - BIS
  - If needed:
    - Arterial line
    - Central venous pressure (CVP)

23. Common Adult Setup at Teaching Hospitals

Pre-Medication:

- midazolam (3 ml syringe)

Induction Medication:

- propofol or etomidate (20 ml syringe)
    - Only one is drawn up — don't pull a rookie mistake and draw up both.

Induction Adjuncts:

- fentanyl (5 ml syringe)
- lidocaine (5 ml syringe)
    - Lidocaine is used to reduce the pain on injection of propofol.

Neuromuscular Blockers:

- Usually only one is drawn up.
- If you are doing a rapid sequence induction, then draw up succinylcholine and one of the following should be used.
    - succinylcholine (10 ml syringe)
    - vecuronium (10 ml syringe)
    - rocuronium (5 ml syringe)
    - cisatracurium (10 ml syringe)

Neuromuscular Reversals:

- Some staff members prefer to have you draw these up at the end of the case so that they are not accidentally used during the case.
    - glycopyrrolate (5 ml syringe)
    - neostigmine (5 ml syringe)

Antiemetic Medications:

- dexamethasone (3 ml syringe) — to be given at the start of the case

- ondansetron (3 ml syringe) — to be given at the end of the case

Adrenergic Medications:

- ephedrine (10 ml) — requires a single dilution (see ch. 13)
- phenylephrine (10 ml) — requires a double dilution (see ch. 13)

Table 16 The Typical Setup		
	Medication	Syringe Size
Preop		
	midazolam	3 ml
Intraop		
	propofol*	20 ml
	etomidate*	20 ml
	fentanyl	5 ml
	morphine	5 ml
	lidocaine	5 ml
	succinylchoine	10 ml
	vecuronium**	10 ml
	rocuronium**	5 ml
	cisatracurium**	10 ml
Reversals		
	glycopyrrolate	5 ml
	neostigmine	5 ml
PONV		
	dexamethazone	3 ml
	ondansetron	3 ml
* draw up only propofol or etomidate, not both		
** only draw up one paralytic		

24. Adult Airway Management

Perhaps you are doing an airway rotation or an "anesthesia rotation" just to get experience managing airways. There are a few things that can make your experience more useful.

Before you start your rotation, read through this chapter and have someone show you how to do these skills on a mannequin or watch some YouTube vides to see how it is done. Airway skills require the three *p*'s: patience, patients, and practice.

When someone is showing you these skills in the OR, pay close attention to each step.

Don't worry about speed when you are starting. Get the mechanics down and the speed will come. Remember: "Slow is smooth ... Smooth is Fast."

There is nothing worse than traumatizing an airway and causing bleeding by being too aggressive. Keep a constant flow of communication between you and your staff to let them know what you feel and see: "The patient is easy to mask." "I see the epiglottis." "The tube is passing through the vocal cords."

Basic Airway Anatomy:

- nasopharynx
  - The nasal airway from the nose to the soft palate.
- oropharynx
  - The oral airway from the soft palate to the epiglottis.
- hypopharynx
  - The airway from the epiglottis to the esophagus.
- larynx
  - Inlet to the trachea and lungs
- trachea
  - Extends from the larynx to the carina.

Equipment for Airway Management:

SALT

S - suction (most commonly forgotten piece of equipment)

A - airway (oral airway)

L - laryngoscope

T - tube (endotracheal tube)

(in the OR, what kind

(clearing)

The Brief Airway History

You will want to get a brief history from the patient or bystanders to help you with the airway management. You can use the $W^2A^2S^2$ acronym. Think of it as "Why *was* I called to the bedside of this patient?" $W^2A^2S^2$

- W - why called to bedside (in the OR, what kind of airway is going to be placed)
- W - weight of the patient
- A - age of the patient
- A - allergies
- S - significant past medical history
- S - stomach — when was the last meal?

The 4 Basic Airway Skills

There are four basic airway skills you should work on during your airway rotation:

1. Mask ventilation
2. Laryngeal mask airway (LMA) placement
3. Intubation
4. Confirmation that your LMA or ETT is properly placed and working

Adult Patient Flow

It is helpful to know what to expect when on an airway rotation. For adult patients, they will have an IV in place and will usually have already received an anxiolysis before coming to the OR.

They will be moved over to the OR table (when you help with the patient transfer, make sure both the OR table and the patient stretcher are locked). Once on the OR table, the patient will have monitors attached, will have one final pre-induction set of vitals taken, and will be pre-oxygenated. The anesthesia team member you are working with will then give the patient medications to induce the patient into general anesthesia. At this point, the anesthetist will have you take over the airway and have you mask ventilate the patient. It is from here on out that you will be managing the patient's airway.

Mask Ventilation

This is the most important skill to learn during your rotation. If you can efficiently mask ventilate your patient, you can buy time to think, get help, and set up equipment.

Select the proper size mask: chin lift / jaw thrust.

• Think of mask ventilation as bringing the jaw up to the mask, not the mask being pushed down on the face.

Provide enough positive pressure to have the chest rise.

• Try to limit your pressure to below 20 cm H2O.

• Airway gastric pressure above 20 cm H2O can open the patient's lower esophageal sphincter and cause gastric distention.

• If you overfill the lungs, the air goes into the stomach and can cause distention.

• Enough distention and you increase the risk of

• difficulty ventilating or

• passive stomach regurgitation.

Mask Ventilation Adjuncts:
Oropharyngeal airway (OPA)

- Measured from corner of the mouth to angle of the jaw
- Can cause gagging/vomiting if the gag reflex is in place
- Avoid placing while the patient is in Stage 2 of anesthesia (see ch. 4) if possible to avoid laryngospasm

Nasopharyngeal airway (NPA)

- Measured from the naris to the angle of the jaw
- Does not affect gag reflex
- Can cause epistaxis (bloody nose)
    - Pretreat the nose with a topical vasoconstrictor (oxymetazoline) and use a liquid lubricant on the NPA to minimize trauma.

Confirmation of Mask Ventilation:

- Chest rise
- Breath sounds
- EtCO2

LMA Placement

This device is a "mask," but it "sits" in the back of the pharynx, over the airway.
It is placed blindly (you are not directly looking where the device is going) and can be a good rescue airway device.

The LMA is not a "secured" airway because if the patient passively (or actively) regurgitates, the stomach contents can go into the "bowl" of the LMA and be directed into the trachea, and ultimately into the lungs.

There are many different types of LMAs; however, most have the same basic shape.

1. Select the proper size based on weight (see chart below).
   - Each LMA package should have the weight range printed on the package.
2. Open the package and lightly lubricate the device.
3. With the patient's head in the neutral position, open the mouth.
4. Place the LMA against the hard palate and gently advance the device until gentle resistance is felt.
   - At this point the LMA should "seat" itself around the airway.
5. Inflate the LMA
   - Many times the LMA will back slightly out as it "seats" in the airway.
6. Attach the LMA to your breathing circuit.
7. Confirm the placement of LMA with one gentle breath through the bag apparatus.
   - Chest rise
   - Breath sounds
   - EtCO2
8. Secure the LMA with tape.

Intubation

This is the gold standard for securing the patient's airway. It protects the airway from secretions, blood, and stomach contents. Intubation also allows for positive pressure ventilation without the risk of gastric distention. The most important skill is to be able to confirm proper placement of an ETT.

Prepare Your Equipment:
- Make sure your SALT is working
- Select the properly sized equipment
  - Laryngoscope blades come in two basic types:
    - Straight (most common is called Miller)
    - Curved (most common is Macintosh, or Mac for short.)
  - Depending on body habitus/weight, most adult patients will be intubated with either a Miller 2 or 3 laryngoscope or a Macintosh 3 or 4 laryngoscope.
  - Select a size 7.0 endotracheal tube (ETT) for most women, and an 8.0 ETT for most men.

Prepare the Patient

Position the patient at the head of the bed. Raise the height of the bed until the patient's head is at the height of your xiphoid process.
- Place a small pillow under the patient's head to provide anterior alignment of the head.
- An intubation pillow will help to align the airway to see the vocal cords.
- Make sure you have a good mask seal and you can ventilate the patient.

Prepare Yourself:
- The laryngoscope handle is held in your left hand.
  - It does not matter whether you are right- or left-handed.
- Have someone hold your ETT.

• The suction will go next to your right hand.

Oral Intubation:

1. Remove the mask.

2. Gently tilt the head back, and open the mouth with your right hand.

3. Use your left hand to gently place the laryngoscope blade in the patient's mouth.

    • Start at the right side of the mouth and use the blade of the laryngoscope to sweep the tongue to the left side.

4. Continue to advance the blade deeper into the patient's airway and you will see

    1. the palate and tongue,

    2. then the epiglottis, and

    3. as you lift the epiglottis using anterior pressure, you will start to see airway structures.

    • Adjust your view, until you have the best possible view.

    • Never use the teeth as a fulcrum.

    • The vector of your laryngoscope pressure should be as if the handle of the laryngoscope is being lifted straight up.

5. Grade your view without cricoid pressure and with cricoid pressure (if needed).

    • Grade 1 - full view of the vocal cords

    • Grade 2A - partial view of the vocal cords

    • Grade 2B - only the arytenoids and epiglottis visible

    • Grade 3 - only epiglottis visible

- Grade 4 - neither the epiglottis nor glottis visible

6. Using your right hand, introduce the ETT at the right side of the mouth and advance it through the airway.
7. Watch as the ETT passes between the vocal cords and make sure the cuff of the ETT is past the vocal cords.
8. Hold the ETT in place with your right hand and gently remove the laryngoscope blade.
   - Make sure you don't touch the teeth while removing the scope.
9. Continue to hold the ETT in place until it is taped.

Confirmation of Orally Placed ETT:
- Chest rise with ventilation
- "Fog" in the ETT with expiration
- Bilateral breath sounds present
- No sounds over the stomach
- Sustained EtCO2 (gold standard)

Nasal Intubation

In addition to standard intubation equipment, you will also need Magill forceps.

Some anesthesia providers also use a nasal RAE (a special ETT with a non-kinking bend).

1. Prepare the nose
   - Many times, you will be preparing the nose while continuing to give positive pressure ventilation to the patient, after he or she is asleep. Use either lubricant

and/or nasally placed topical vasoconstrictor (to reduce bleeding).

- Some dilate the nose with nasopharyngeal airways (NPA—aka nasal trumpets), whereas others use a red rubber catheter to reduce the trauma to the nasal mucosa.

2. Place the ETT through the nares

- Gently pass the ETT through the nose, either with or without the use of a red rubber catheter.
- The laryngoscope is then placed in the mouth as you would for an oral intubation.
- Grasp the ETT with the Magill forceps, being careful not to tear the ETT cuff.

3. The vocal cords are then visualized as with an oral intubation.

4. Guide the ETT between the vocal cords.

5. Confirm the placement of the ETT as described above.

If the patient starts to desaturate during the nasal intubation attempt, you have to stay cool. You have two options:

1. Remove the laryngoscope/ETT and mask ventilate the patient.

- This can cause bleeding from the nose to pool in the oropharynx.
- Once the SpO2 has improved, reinitiate your intubation attempt.

2. Pull the ETT back so that it is above the larynx and

   - remove the laryngoscope,
   - manually close the mouth,
   - pinch the naris closed that doesn't have the ETT in it,
   - gently ventilate the patient until you get chest rise, and
   - once the SpO2 has improved, reinitiate your intubation attempt.

Confirmation of Nasally Placed ETT:

- Chest rise with inspiration
- "Fog" in the ETT with expiration
- Breath sounds present
- No sounds over the stomach
- Sustained EtCO2 (gold standard)

Nasal Intubation Caveat:

Nasal intubation is usually done for surgery involving the oral cavity, mandible, or floor of the mouth. It is routine for the surgeons to place a throat pack in the back of the pharynx before they start operating to keep blood and secretions from filling the stomach. At the end of surgery, it is vital to have the surgeons remove the throat pack when they are done with the surgery. If the throat pack is left in the mouth, and the patient is extubated, then the pack can cause airway obstruction. **This is a potentially lethal mistake when the surgeons are wiring the jaw closed!**

When the surgeons are done, or just before they start to wire the jaw closed, double-check that the throat pack has been removed. If the jaw is wired closed, make sure wire cutters go with the patient to the PACU so you can open the jaw in an emergency.

Parting Words to the Airway Rotator, New Anesthesia Student, or Resident
Although masking the patient may not seem "exciting" to you, it is vital that you learn this skill. You're on your rotation to learn airway management, not just intubations. Having the ability to mask ventilate the patient can buy you, and the patient, time. There are multiple times that I have rescued patients because I could mask ventilate properly. I have also saved patients by placing an LMA or intubating when someone else could not. Having all these skills will allow you to better manage airways when they are straightforward and also when they become challenging and difficult.

When you are in a challenging airway case, don't forget to breathe for the patient and breathe for yourself. Smooth is fast. Learn the mechanics and speed will come.

25. Pediatric Airway Management

Please read chapter 24, "Adult Airway Management," as this information will bolster the information found within this chapter.

Pediatric patients can be more challenging than adult patients. There are a number of differences between pediatric and adult patients, including cardiac, respiratory, renal, liver, and endocrine physiology. Likewise, management of the pediatric airway is also different, even if the basic concepts are still the same.

Airway anatomy differences between adults and pediatric patients.

Pediatric airways are different because:

1. They have a smaller airway (most obvious)
   - The infant's airway diameter can be estimated by the diameter of the patient's pinky finger.
   - The narrowest part of the airway is at the cricoid ring.
     - Just because the ETT can pass through the vocal cords, it does not mean it will "fit" the patient.
   - Small amounts of edema (swelling) can cause big problems because it can decrease the area of the tracheal opening dramatically.
2. Their tongue is larger in comparison to the size of the mouth.
3. Their larynx is anatomically more cephalic (closer to the head).
   - Some mistakenly call it "more anterior."
4. Their epiglottis is shorter and narrower.

Pediatric physiology that affects airway management.
Cardiac/Respiratory

- Increased O2 consumption per kg compared to adults.
  - Infants have twice the O2 consumption per kg compared to adults.
- This causes a rapid desaturation with interruption of ventilation compared to adults.
- With decreases in SpO2, pediatric patients are more prone to bradycardia.
- Increased CO2 production compared to adults.

Therefore, the pediatric patient will desaturate and decompensate quicker than an adult.

When pediatric patients desaturate, they become bradycardic much faster than adults due to their immature parasympathetically driven cardiac physiology. Unless an airway is established, and ventilation and oxygenation occur, then your patient's HR will slow until asystole. This can happen much faster than an adult, so you will need to move quickly to establish an airway.

Some pediatric anesthesiologists have Sux and Atropine drawn up in 3 ml syringes and ready to go with a sharp needle (not plastic) in place should they need to establish an airway in an emergency. It is also handy to have an alcohol prep pad with your syringes (with the patient's weight written on it) so that you can give the medication intramuscularly and you don't have to look for an alcohol prep pad or the patient's weight.

Pediatric Patient Flow

If you are doing a pediatric airway rotation with an anesthesia department, the patient will usually be NPO. For elective pediatric surgery, there is a progression from when the patient is brought into the room until they are ready for you to manage the airway. Knowing the flow of pediatric patients from the holding area to your OR will help you know what to expect.

Typically, the patient will have received premedication to help with separation anxiety from his or her parents, or the parents will accompany the patient to the OR.

Once in the OR, the patient will undergo a mask induction, followed by IV placement, after he or she is asleep. It is important that the patient is through Stage 2 of anesthesia (see ch. 4) before the IV is attempted because of the risk of laryngospasm (see "laryngospasm" below.) Once the IV is placed, then the airway can be instrumented with either an LMA or ETT.

Let's go through each part in more detail.

Anxiety in children can be managed several ways:

1. The patient may be too young to have parental separation issues, so nothing is needed. Some patients start to get separation anxiety at six to nine months of age. Each patient is a little different.
2. One of the patient's parents accompanies the patient to the OR for the mask induction.
3. The patient receives a premedication of either:
   - 0.5 mg/kg midazolam PO or
   - mg/kg midazolam IV
4. A combination of #2 and #3

OR Time

Once in the room, monitors will be placed and the patient will undergo a mask induction with O2 or N2O/O2 in Sevoflourne. You will see the patient go through stage 1 (sedation), stage 2 (excitation), and then to stage 3—general anesthesia (see ch. 4, "Stages of Anesthesia.")

Once the patient is in stage 3, an IV will be started. It is around this time that the patient's airway may be handed over to you.

Prior to assuming the airway, you should do the following:

1. Ask the "W^{2}A^{2}S^2" questions:

W - what kind of airway is going to be placed

W - weight of the patient

A - age of the patient

A - allergies

S - significant past medical history

S - Stomach—full or empty

2. Check SALT

S - suction

A - airway (properly sized OPA or LMA)

L - laryngoscope (properly working)

T - ETT

- Even if the LMA/laryngoscope/ETT size is decided for you, part of your training should be to learn how to calculate and select the properly sized equipment.

For Infants, also consider PAT:

> P – Positioning. They will need a shoulder roll instead of an intubating pillow because of their large head.
>
> A – Atropine. Pretreated with atropine (10 mcg/kg) to maintain the HR should the patient desaturate quickly during the intubation.
>
> T - Tube. An extra ETT that is one size smaller should the selected size not fit.

Sizing Your Equipment

It is helpful to select the proper ETT size you think you need and also prepare a half size smaller in case the larger ETT does not go easily or you do not have an adequate leak (see below).

- Term Neonate
  - Miller 1 blade
  - 3.0 and 3.5 ETT (uncuffed)
- 0–8 months
  - Miller 1 blade
  - 3.5 and 4.0 ETT (uncuffed)
- 8 months–2 years
  - Miller 1 or Macintosh 2 blade
  - 4.0 and 4.5 ETT (uncuffed)
- 2 years–6 years
  - Miller 2 or Macintosh 2 blade
  - use the formula (age/4) +4 for the ETT
- 6–12 years
  - Miller 2 or Macintosh 3 blade
  - ETT (uncuffed) according to the formula (age/4) +4

If you use a cuffed ETT, then choose your uncuffed ETT and downsize by a half size. For example, if you calculate an uncuffed 5.0 ETT, then use a cuffed 4.5 ETT.

The 3 Basic Pediatric Airway Skills

Much like the adult airway rotation, the three basic airway skills are ventilation, LMA placement, and intubation. The skills are similar, but there are some pearls that will make your airway skills, and your rotation, more successful.

Pediatric Mask Ventilation Pearls:

• Properly sized mask and equipment is key.
  • Make sure the mask does not put pressure on the patient's eyes.
• Keep the tongue off the roof of the mouth.
  • This can be done by slightly opening the patient's mouth.
• Sometimes a shoulder roll can help with alignment of the airway, much like you use an intubation pillow for adult patients.
• Give just enough ventilation pressure to get chest rise.
  • If you over-inflate the lungs, the extra air will inflate the stomach.
  • This is even easier to do with pediatric patients, compared to adults.
  • As the stomach becomes larger, it becomes harder to ventilate.
• There are times when an orogastric tube (OGT) may need to be placed, the stomach decompressed, and have the OGT removed to help with ventilation.

LMA Placement Pearls:

- Pediatric placement of LMAs is the same as for adults (see ch. 24, "Adult Airway Management").
- Properly sizing the LMA for the pediatric patient is important and is based on the patient's weight.

If a patient is between LMA sizes, look at the size of the mouth to determine the proper size of the LMA.

Table 15 LMA Sizing

LMA Size	Ideal Patient Weight
#1	< 5 kg
#1.5	5–10 kg
#2	10–20 kg
#2.5	20–30 kg
#3	30–50 kg
#4	50–70 kg
#5	70–100 kg

Pediatric Intubation Pearls:

- Remember, you can always fall back on your mask ventilation skills if you run into problems. Stop trying to intubate, mask ventilate the patient, and buy yourself some time.
- If at any time during your intubation attempt the patient desaturates and the SpO_2% nears 92%, stop your intubation, and mask ventilate the patient with 100% O_2.
- When the attending tells you to stop, then stop.

- You might be "just right there," but there may be "badness" going on and your tunnel vision doesn't see it.
- Some anesthesiologists will premedicate infants with 10 mcg/kg atropine to prevent bradycardia, in case the intubation attempt takes longer than expected.
- A properly sized laryngoscope and ETT at the start of the procedure goes a long way.

Confirmation of ETT Placement:

- Chest rise with inspiration
- "Fog" in the ETT with expiration
- Breath sounds present
- No sounds over the stomach
- EtCO2 (gold standard)

After Confirmation of ETT Placement:

- ETT proper sizing is confirmed with a leak test in pediatric patients.
  - With the ETT in place, the pop-off valve is partially closed to allow pressure to build in the airway.
  - You listen for the escape of air around the ETT and the trachea.
  - Most recommend an audible leak of 15 to 20 cm H2O to prevent tracheal ischemia from an ETT that is too large for the patient.
    - If it is < 10 cm H2O or > 25 cm H2O, the ETT may need to be switched out.

Parting Words

When things go wrong in pediatric anesthesia, they go wrong quickly. Pediatric patients do not have the same amount of reserve for badness that adults do. Respect the patient and the airway. Be gentle when instrumenting the airway; small amounts of edema from rough handling can compromise the airway. Use the minimal force necessary to manage the airway.

If things do go sideways, stay cool, and speak up to your staff or preceptor. Just like with adults, continue to let your staff know what you feel and see.

Laryngospasm

Laryngospasm occurs when there is stimulus of the patient or the airway without enough anesthesia. We tend to see this more commonly in pediatric patients because of mask inductions and deep extubations in this patient population.

A typical scenario involves a patient going through stage 2 when some oral secretions fall on the vocal cords and cause the entire entrance to the trachea to close in on itself. When a laryngospasm occurs, you need to work quickly.

1. Provide continuous positive airway pressure (CPAP) to the patient via the mask with 100% O_2.
2. Provide a jaw thrust or pressure on the laryngospasm notch (anterior to the mastoid process) to help break the laryngospasm.
3. If you have an IV, you can give the patient 0.5 mg/kg of propofol.
4. If you don't have an IV, you can give 2 mg/kg of IM Sux.

26. Advanced Airways

During your rotation, you may also see some advanced airway procedures.

Get good at the standard intubation techniques, and then try some of the techniques below. You will want to use some of the advanced airway devices on some of your standard cases. You don't want to try these devices for the first time when there is an emergency. There is a learning curve for using all these devices, and you should be comfortable with the technique before trying to rely on it in an emergency.

Video Laryngoscopes:

- These laryngoscopes utilize a small camera and a screen (either on the device or attached to it).
- You place the video laryngoscope in the patient's mouth as you would for a standard laryngoscope.
- Instead of looking in the mouth directly, you look at the video screen.
- Note that the video laryngoscope is made with a more acute angle than a standard laryngoscope blade so that you can "see around the corner." Therefore, it is important to use an ETT with a stylet and put the same angle bend in it as the video laryngoscope blade.
- The ETT is then placed in the mouth, and you guide it to the airway indirectly while looking at the screen.
- Glidescope™, McGrath™, and Truview™ are three examples of such devices.

Fiber-Optic Scopes:

- These airway devices use a flexible fiber-optic cable with a camera and a light source on the end to guide the ETT through the vocal cords.
- Usually the ETT is placed over the fiber-optic scope, and then you place the scope through the nose or mouth.
- Once the fiber-optic scope is placed through the vocal cords, the ETT is then slid over the scope until it is through the cords.

Others

There tend to be new airway devices introduced every year. Most are variations on one of the themes above. The two most common types, as described above, are what you will more than likely encounter on an anesthesia rotation. If you have the opportunity to try a new device, do so. However, your focus should be on mastering direct laryngoscopy with a laryngoscope. These devices will not be available throughout the hospital, so you will need to become proficient with the direct laryngoscopy.

27. Rapid Sequence Induction (RSI)

An RSI is used when the patient isn't NPO (has a full stomach), is actively vomiting, or has an aspiration risk due to an underlying condition. The goal is to put the patient to sleep quickly, relax his or her muscles so that he or she cannot actively vomit, and place the ETT in the trachea to secure the airway. Most people use a rapid acting induction agent along with a paralytic drug.

Drugs commonly used for RSI:
- Propofol (2 mg/kg) or etomidate (0.2 mg/kg)
    - Propofol is used for hemodynamically stable patients
    - Etomidate is used for hemodynamically unstable patients
- Succinylcholine (1 mg/kg)
- Rocuronium (1.2 mg/kg)
    - For those who have a contraindication to Sux

RSI example:
- Prepare all your SALT equipment.
    - You might also want to prepare an orogastric tube to empty out the stomach once you secure the airway.
- Pre-oxygenate with 100% O2
    - This is done to try to keep the patient oxygenated during the intubation attempt.
- Rapidly push IV medications
    - 2 mg/kg of propofol followed quickly by
    - 1 mg/kg succynolcholine

- Orally intubate the patient.
- Confirm intubation as described in chapters 24 and 25.

Historically, cricoid pressure was used in an effort to prevent passive regurgitation of stomach contents. However, this technique seems to have fallen out of favor because there is not enough data to support its effectiveness to continue to practice the technique.

RSI Pearls:

- Smooth is fast

- Prepare all your equipment and have your suction available, and be prepared to turn the patient on his or her left side if vomiting occurs.

- If vomiting does occur, by rotating the patient onto his or her left side, you can then intubate the patient.

- If you are using succinylcholine, wait until the patient has stopped fasciculating (the involuntary muscle jerking) and relaxes before attempting to open the patient's mouth to intubate.

- If you are using rocuronium, make sure you wait long enough before attempting to intubate. Usually 90 seconds is long enough.

- Some staff may have you put the patient in reverse Trendelenburg (head up) with a tilt of 10–15 degrees to help with passive regurgitation.

28. Putting It All Together—A Case Example

You are told that you will be providing anesthesia for a 30 y/o female who is undergoing an emergent laparoscopic appendectomy (Lap Appy).

Pre-Op:

You complete your anesthesia H&P:

- She has no past medical history.
- Her vital signs are within normal limits.
- Weight: 70 kg
- She ate right before she came into the hospital 1 hour ago.

Physical Exam:

- Airway exam: MP I, 3 finger breadths thyromental distance, and good neck extension.
- Heart: RRR without murmur
- Lungs: CTA bilaterally
- Urine pregnancy test is negative
- She has an 18 gauge IV in her left hand and is nervous during the H&P.

Your Anesthetic Plan:

ASA 1E patient for a "lap appy". You will be doing a general anesthetic with rapid sequence induction (RSI) on an otherwise healthy patient. She is at risk for PONV because she is a nonsmoker, female, and has a history of motion sickness.

You set up your room:

- Positioning - no special positioning is needed
- Machine check - done
- Suction - operational
- Monitors - standard monitors are in place and operational
- Airway - Mac 3 laryngoscope blade and 7.0 cuffed ETT

- IV equipment - the patient already has an IV, but you have an IV bag and tubing set up.
- Drugs
    - Midazolam 2 mg (3 ml syringe)
    - 1% Lidocaine 5 ml (5 ml syringe)
    - Propofol 200 mg (20 ml syringe)
    - Fentanyl 500 mcg (5 ml syringe)
    - Succinylcholine 200 mg (10 ml syringe)
    - Vecuronium 10 mg (10 ml syringe)
    - Neosynephrine (100 mcg/ml after double dilution - 10 ml syringe)
    - Ephedrine (5 mg/ml after single dilution - 10 ml syringe)
- Special - You have your seat, and you don't need anything special.

Induction:

- You give the patient 2 mg IV midazolam in the preoperative suite and bring the patient to the OR.
- You place monitors on the patient, take a new BP in the OR, and start to preoxygenate the patient.
- You wait until the attending anesthesiologist is in the room, and then you begin your induction.
You decide to give the following:
- 150 mcg of fentanyl (3 ml given)
- 50 mg of lidocaine (5 ml given)
- 150 mg propofol (15 ml given)
- 70 mg of succinylcholine (7 ml given)

You wait until the patient has stopped fasciculating and is relaxed, and then you intubate the patient.

Once the ETT cuff is up, you see "fog" in the ETT, breath sounds are present, you see $EtCO_2$ on your monitor, and then you secure the ETT and start the ventilator. You place a bite block to keep the patient from occluding the ETT when she is waking up at the end of the case during emergence.

You dial in 6% desflurane slowly over several breaths, so you don't cause tachycardia.

You adjust your fresh gas flows to 1L O_2 and 1L air. You check the patient's paralysis with a twitch monitor on the patient's ulnar nerve and see that twitches have returned; you then give 4 mg of vecuronium. You also give 4 mg of dexamethasone for PONV prevention and settle into the case. You also place an orogastric tube (OGT), attached it to low wall suction to empty any stomach contents that are present.

Maintenance of Anesthesia

While the patient is being prepped by the circulator nurse, you notice that with the full anesthetic in place and no surgical stimulation, the patient's BP is starting to down trend.

The patient has a high HR and a down trending BP, so you give her 50 mcg phenylephrine (0.5 ml given), which she responds to nicely—her HR starts to slow and when the next BP is taken, you see that her BP has come back up. The surgery continues without further incident.

Throughout the rest of the case, you give boluses of 25 mcg of fentanyl (0.5 ml at a time) in response to increased HR and BP. Toward the end of the case, you draw up your reversal medications:

- 5 mg of neostigmine (5 ml syringe)
- 1 mg of glycopyrrolate (5 ml syringe)

You start to titrate in some morphine 2 mg x 2. As the surgeons are finishing up, you start planning your landing.

Emergence from Anesthesia

You give 4 mg of ondansetron as part of your PONV prevention plan.

You decrease the respiratory rate and/or tidal volume on the ventilator to allow the $EtCO_2$ to get higher so that she will start to breathe on her own. You place the OGT on active wall suction one last time and remove the tube, being careful not to extubate the patient.

You start "dialing down" the vaporizer to reduce the vapor and continue to do so throughout emergence.

When the fascial layer of the abdominal wall is sutured closed, you check twitches, and seeing that you have at least one twitch, you give full reversal:

- 5 mg of neostigmine (5 ml) and 1 mg of glycopyrrolate (5 ml)

You turn off the ventilator when the patient is starting to breathe spontaneously. You titrate in more morphine to reduce the respiratory rate to around 10 breaths/min. Turn the vaporizer off and let the rest of the vapor be "blown off" by the patient.

The patient's port sites are now closed, bandages applied, and the surgery is complete. When the patient is awake, swallowing, and following commands, you deflate the ETT cuff and extubate the patient. You bring the patient to the PACU, give report to the PACU RN, and finish up your paperwork. You then get ready for the next case.

29. Regional Anesthesia

Regional anesthesia is the placement of local anesthesia around nerves to numb regions of the patient's body. We also place the local anesthesia around a bundle of nerves (usually under ultrasound guidance) that will localize the area of the body we want to numb up.

There are several different types of regional anesthesia that you may encounter, either as the sole anesthetic or in combination with general anesthesia. If you need to dilute the medications, be sure to use preservative-free solutions so as to not cause potential nerve damage from the preservative.

Table 13 Common Local Anesthetics			
Local Anesthesia	Max Dose Plain	Max Dose with Epi	Onset
bupivacaine	2.5 mg/kg	3 mg/kg	5–15 min.
lidocaine	4.5 mg/kg	7 mg/kg	5–15 min.
ropivacaine	2.5 mg/kg	2.5 mg/kg	10–20 min.

Peripheral Nerve Block

These "blocks" are used either for surgery or postoperative pain control. You use external landmarks, a stimulator needle, or ultrasound to find the nerves you want to block. You then guide the needle to a location close to the nerves and deliver local anesthetic to the area to bathe nerves and block the transmission of pain impulses.

Peripheral nerve blocks can be done for a variety of locations, but perhaps most commonly, they are used for upper/lower extremity surgery.

Epidural

With epidural anesthesia, a needle is placed in the patient's back and advanced between the spinous processes to the epidural space. A small catheter is then placed into the space and local anesthesia is injected to bathe the nerves in this area. The location of entry of the epidural catheter (from the lumbar spine to the cervical spine) and the volume of local anesthetic used will determine what level of analgesia will be provided. **When an epidural is placed, the needle will pass through the following:**

- skin
- subcutaneous tissue
- supraspinous ligament
- interspinous ligament (when the needle is firmly embedded here, it will maintain it's angle when the operator lets go of the needle)
- ligamentum flavum
- epidural space

- And if it advances too far, dura, which will lead to a "wet tap" when you have cerebral spinal fluid (CSF) gush out your needle.

What this will look like when you see someone place an epidural:

1. This is a sterile procedure.
    - Once the operator puts on sterile gloves, he or she will have to make sure not to contaminate him- or herself or the sterile field.
2. The patient's back will be cleaned with a sterile solution (usually betadine), a sterile drape is placed over the entire back, and the excess solution is wiped away.
3. The operator will place some local anesthetic in the entry point of the epidural with a small needle to
    1. numb the patient and
    2. to find the angle of projection toward the epidural space.
4. A larger Tuohy needle is then placed and advanced through the first 4 layers, until it is embedded in the interspinous ligament
5. The stylet is then removed from the needle.
6. A syringe with either air or sterile saline is placed on the Tuohy.
7. The Tuohy with the syringe is then advanced while either giving continuous or intermittent "pressure" on the plunger of the syringe.
8. The apparatus is advanced until a "loss of resistance" is felt and the plunger is able to inject either the air or water.

- This is how the epidural space is found.

9. The operator notes the markings on the needle to determine how deep the needle was placed.

10. The syringe is removed, and a catheter is placed through the Tuohy needle and threaded into the epidural space.

    - Always advance the catheter through the needle.
    - Never pull the catheter back through the needle, or the catheter can be sheared off.

11. Length markings on the epidural catheter are noted, and then the needle is completely removed from the back.

    - Pull back until there is about 3 to 4 cm of catheter in the epidural space.

12. An adaptor with a Luer Lock is then placed on the end of the catheter so that a standard syringe can be attached to the catheter and medications can be pushed through the catheter.

13. The epidural catheter is then tested with a solution of lidocaine with epinephrine.

    - 3 ml of 1.5% lidocaine with 1:200,000 epinephrine
    - This "test dose" checks for
        1. intrathecal placement (if the catheter was there, the patient would get a profound block), and

2. intravascular placement (the patient could have headache, oral numbness, blurry vision, or ringing in the ears) or tachycardia from the Epi.

14. Once the test dose is negative, then the epidural is dosed with local anesthesia for either analgesia or for surgery.

15. A clear occlusive dressing is placed over the site of the epidural so that the markings of the epidural can be seen to indicate the depth of insertion.

    • Tape is then placed over the rest of the epidural catheter to further secure it.

Caudal

With this technique, which is typically used in infants and children, the medication is placed in the same place as an epidural (the epidural space); however, the space is accessed by way of a needle or IV catheter through the sacral hiatus, which is located close to the tailbone. The sacral hiatus, which is covered by the sacrococcygeal ligament, tends to calcify after childhood, which makes placing a caudal in adults difficult.

What you will observe.

Typically, caudals are placed on infants and children after they are under general anesthesia.

1. Using a sterile technique and gloves, the patient's back will be prepped.

2. The patient is placed on his or her side.

3. The area is cleaned and a sterile drape is placed.

4. The sacral hiatus is palpated with a sterile gloved hand.
5. A needle or IV catheter is then placed through the ligament that runs between the cornua of the sacrum at a 45% angle.
6. The needle or IV catheter is advanced slowly until resistance "gives."
7. The needle/IV catheter is then flattened and advanced slightly parallel to the patient's body.

> • If a blunt tipped is being used,
>   1. then you attach your syringe of local,
>   2. draw back to make sure you are not in the CSF, and
>   3. then slowly inject.
>
> • If an IV catheter is being used,
>   1. then advance the catheter,
>   2. attach a syringe, draw back, and
>   3. then slowly inject.

Spinal

This technique places the medication within the dura, where the cerebral spinal fluid resides. The procedure will be similar to an epidural, but only a thin needle will be used instead of the larger Tuohy needle and confirmation of proper placement of the needle is with a return of cerebral spinal fluid (CSF) through the end of the needle.

What you will observe.

1. This is a sterile procedure.
   - Once the operator puts on sterile gloves, he or she will have to make sure not to contaminate him- or herself or the sterile field.
2. The patient's back will be cleaned with a sterile solution (usually betadine), a sterile drape is placed over the entire back, and the excess solution is wiped away.
3. The operator will infiltrate some local anesthetic with a small needle
   - to numb the patient and
   - to find the angle of projection toward the subdural space.
4. An introducer needle will be placed in the patients back.
5. A longer, thinner needle will be placed through the introducer and advanced until a "pop" is felt.
6. The stylet is then removed from the needle and the needle is stabilized. The stylet is not discarded.
7. CSF should be seen dripping from the end of the needle.
8. The spinal medication syringe is then attached to the spinal needle.
9. The plunger is pulled gently back to see the mixing of the CSF with the local mixture.
10. The medication is administered and the syringe is removed from the needle.
11. The stylet is replaced, and the introducer and spinal needle are removed at the same time.

12. Sterile gauze is then held over the needle site with gentle pressure until a bandage can be placed.

Regional Technique Resources

You need to see some of these types of procedures to fully appreciate them. One of the best websites available is the New York School of Regional Anesthesia at www.nysora.com. There are free resources on how to do nerve blocks and videos that show you the anatomy used to place the block.

30. Obstetric Anesthesia

During your introduction to anesthesiology, you may be placed on an obstetric (OB) anesthesia rotation. During this rotation, you will hone some skills that will serve you well in the OB delivery rooms, the OB surgical suite, and in the general OR.

There are whole textbooks written on OB anesthesia. I will outline the basic survival skills to get you going on the rotation.

Physiologic Changes of Pregnancy

Your pregnant patient will undergo changes even early on in pregnancy. As the pregnancy progresses, providing safe anesthesia care will become more challenging.

Neurologic Changes

MAC requirements: Pregnant patients have a decreased MAC compared to nonpregnant patients. This is good to keep in mind when providing general anesthesia to these patients.

Considerations for epidurals/spinals: Because of gravid uterus, the enlarged epidural veins lead to a decrease in both the epidural space and a relative decease in the volume of CSF. This combination leads to a larger spread of local anesthesia in the near-term patient.

Respiratory Changes

The airway of the pregnant patient becomes more challenging:

1. The airway becomes more friable and easier to be damaged due to changes in the oral mucosal.
2. Intubating the trachea may require a smaller cuffed ETT due to edema of the upper airway.
3. Rapid desaturation can occur during intubation due to
    1. decreased oxygen reserve (decreased functional reserve capacity [FRC] due to the gravid uterus) and
    2. increased oxygen consumption by the mother due to the fetal demands.

The tidal volumes of breathing will increase leading to an increase in minute ventilation.

Cardiovascular Changes

Throughout pregnancy, the patient will have

1. an increasing intravascular fluid volume (of both plasma and red blood cells),
2. an increased cardiac output (CO) — this is caused by both increases in SV and HR; immediately after delivery, the CO can increase up to 80% of baseline —
3. decreasing SVR.

Aortocaval Compression

When the gravid uterus gets large enough, it compresses the mother's inferior vena cava and aorta when the patient is supine. By placing a bump under the supine mother's right hip to raise it about 15 cm, the uterus will be displaced to the left and relieve part of the compression.

Gastrointestinal (GI) Changes

Increased GI reflux occurs in terms of frequency, amount of refluxed stomach contents, and the acidity of contents.

Pregnant patients also have a higher likelihood of having a full stomach because of decreased gut motility and possibly an increased frequency of eating. This puts pregnant patients at risk for pulmonary aspiration, which can further complicate airway manipulation in the patient.

Epidurals for Labor/Delivery Analgesia

Typically, the anesthesia team is called upon to assist with the placement and management of an epidural for labor/delivery analgesia.

Epidurals can be placed, as described in chapter 29, "Regional Anesthesia," with the patient in the seated position. The patient can also be placed in the left lateral position, which tends to be more comfortable for the patient in labor.

Usually an infusion of relatively dilute local anesthesia with/without an opioid is used to provide pain management. Local anesthesia within your epidural solution will numb the nerves in the area that the solution bathes. If opioid is added to the solution, some of it will work at the level of the spinal cord and some will be absorbed systemically and work systemically.

As an epidural is "dosed up," periodically check the level of the epidural by either using ice or a point end of a paperclip to determine the dermatome of the analgesia.

Epidural Complications

Hypotension

Hypotension, the most common complication, is caused by sympathetic nervous system blockade leading to decreased SVR and decreased BP (see ch. 12, "Autonomic Nervous System Medications").

You can pretreat with 250–500 ml of IV fluids to help minimize the problems.
Once the patient is supine, treat with left uterus displacement, more IV fluids if safe to do so, and vasopressors if needed.

High Spinal or High Epidural

This is where the level of the nerves affected by the spinal/epidural is higher than what you intended. This can cause difficulty breathing, unconsciousness, and cardiovascular collapse.

If the patient has a higher spinal or epidural level than what you anticipate, turn down the infusion rate of the epidural and continue to monitor closely. (Also communicate with your staff or preceptor to let him or her know what is going on.)
If the patient has a total spinal, then intubate and support the cardiovascular system. Continue to monitor the fetal heart tones throughout.

Decreased Labor Progress

You may be asked to "turn down" the rate on the epidural infusion to help with the second stage of delivery. Epidurals have been shown to slightly slow the second stage of delivery.

Anesthesia for Caesarean Section (C-Section)

Don't let this common form of delivery fool you. C-sections are "full on" abdominal surgery under regional anesthesia. This is an exciting time for the mother and her family. You have to step up the communications with your patient and the rest of the surgical team. Anticipate problems before they occur.

You must be ready to convert to a general anesthetic should the patient become unstable or if the current regional anesthetic fails. Do a full MS-MAIDS check so that you have the necessary equipment should you need it. Stay cool.

Additional Medications to Prepare for C-Section
- metoclopramide 10 mg IV
- cimetidine 300 mg IV
- sodium citrate 10–30 ml PO
- oxytocin 10 to 40 units after delivery of the placenta

Epidural Anesthesia

If the patient has a good working labor epidural in place, then you can "dose it up." Following a test dose of 3 ml of 2% lidocaine with 1:200,000 epinephrine, you can slowly titrate in 2% lidocaine at 5 ml slow injection into the epidural up to a volume of 20 ml. With each 5 ml increment, check the level of the epidural anesthesia.

Spinal Anesthesia

Spinal anesthesia can be a quick and safe alternative to epidural anesthesia when there may not be time to place an epidural. Some institutions use a combined spinal/epidural whereby they place a Touhy needle, find the loss resistance, and then place a special spinal needle through the Touhy to deliver the spinal anesthesia. This allows for an immediate surgical anesthesia and the placement of an epidural to help with postoperative pain control.

Local Anesthesia

This is a technique in which the surgeons place local anesthesia as they dissect through the abdomen to the uterus to deliver the baby. This technique is typically not done at many institutions anymore, but it can be reserved for patients requiring C-section who are at high risk for general anesthesia and have a contraindication for regional anesthesia.

General Anesthesia

This can be the most controlled and yet the highest risk. The risks involved with the pregnant patient are difficult airway, aspiration, possible fetal depression, and possible awareness under general anesthesia. Much of your prep will center around airway and aspiration precautions.

Prep Your Gear
Standard PMS-MAIDS
Other things to consider:

- Prepare equipment for left uterine displacement.
- midazolam 2 mg IV
- draw up induction dose of
  - propofol 2–2.5 mg/kg (if hemodynamically stable)

    or
  - etomidate 0.2–0.4 mg/kg (if unstable)

- succinylcholine 1 mg/kg
- vecuronium or rocuronium prepared
- fentanyl or morphine ready after delivery of the fetus

Prep the Patient

For aspiration prevention give:

- metoclopramide 10 mg IV (to increase gut motility)
- cimetidine 300 mg IV (to decrease the amount of acid production)
- sodium citrate 10–30 ml PO (to neutralize the acid already in the stomach)

Move the patient to the OR table and place her supine with left uterine displacement. Pre-oxygenate as the patient is being prepped by the surgical team. Have the surgeon/assistants scrubbed in and the patient draped and prepared for delivery before you induce. Continue to talk with the mother throughout the entire episode. This can be one of the most scary times. It is your job to make sure the patient doesn't get "lost" in the rush to deliver the baby.

Have a backup plan for a failed airway.

Good to Go:

Make sure everything is ready: the patient is positioned (with left uterine displacement), draped out, and pre-oxygenated. Put your suction right next to where you need it. Take a breath.

Do a RSI

1. Administer propofol and then succinylcholine when the patient is unconscious.

2. Communicate to the surgeons when ETT placement is confirmed with EtCO2 and the ETT is secured.

3. Quickly turn on 50% N2O and 0.5 MAC of Sevoflurane.
   - This gives you hypnosis without too much Sevo, which can cause relaxation of the uterus.

4. Give vecuronium or rocuronium after return of muscle twitches.

5. Give fentanyl or morphine after the fetus is delivered.

6. Prepare to give oxytocin when the placenta is delivered.

7. Once the baby is delivered, pay attention to any bleeding in the field and the potential for the need to transfuse the patient with blood.

8. The surgeons may ask for you to give methergine to the patient to help with uterine atony. If asked to give methergine, the dose is 0.2 mg (the vial) given IM to the patient's anterior deltoid muscle.

9. If the surgeons ask for you to relax the uterus, increase your Sevo concentration.

10. As the surgeons are closing the abdomen, make your final checks for landing.

11. Remember to reverse the paralytic, give PONV medication, and titrate in your pain medications.

144 / Anesthesia Made Easy

12. Because she is considered a full stomach, wake the patient up when she is ready to be extubated.

OB Anesthesia Pearls

The OB airway is a difficult airway, until proven otherwise.

- Respect the airway . . . but do not be fearful of it.
- Do a very thorough airway exam.
- Use your most experienced person to intubate, not the newest member of the team. This is not the time to "practice" your airways.

The pregnant patient is a full stomach . . . always.

- Part of this is because she may have just eaten and because of hormones of pregnancy.

Place a bump under the patient's right side to displace the uterus off the vena cava and aorta.

- It is more comfortable for her, and it will also help with blood return to the heart.

After placement of an epidural or spinal, watch for hypotension.

- Nausea may be your first sign of hypotension. If she complains of nausea, take another BP and consider giving phenylephrine or ephedrine, depending on the HR and BP. (Some institutions will prefer you use ephedrine.)
- Treat the hypotension and you will treat the nausea.

Learn how to place an epidural while the patient is in the lateral position.

- Place the epidural in the lateral position and dose up the epidural while supine.

- This is more comfortable for mom and expands your techniques.

31. Malignant Hyperthermia

Great resource: Malignant Hyperthermia Association of the United States

http://www.mhaus.org/

For emergencies only:

United States: 1+800-644-9737

Outside the United States: 00+1+209-417-3722

Background

Malignant hyperthermia (MH) is a hypermetabolic state that is triggered in susceptible patients with exposure to volatile anesthetics and succinylcholine. (Air, oxygen, and N2O are safe to use.) It is an inherited disorder that is the result of a mutation in the calcium channel in the skeletal muscle cell. When one of the triggers starts the reaction, calcium is released from within the muscle cell, which causes a hypermetabolic state.

With the metabolic increase within the muscles, the muscles break down, leading to increase in myoglobin in the blood, which can cause renal failure. Ultimately, the patient dies from multiorgan failure if not treated. Even with treatment, the mortality rate is 5–30%

Symptoms include the following:

- muscle rigidity
- tachycardia
- hypertension
- increased EtCO2
- hyperthermia — a very late sign

Preoperative Assessment

Listen for the trigger words while taking the patient and family history:

- "died under general anesthesia"
- "allergic to anesthesia drugs"
- "ran a high fever with anesthesia"
- "woke up in the ICU"
- "woke up packed in ice in the ICU"

When you hear these phrases during your interview, you should ask more questions and try and figure out if it was malignant hyperthermia.

Patients at Risk:

- Patient with central core disease
- Patients with strong family history (see pre-op questions above)
- Patients with certain skeletal muscle disorders (especially pediatric patients)

Prevention in Patients at Risk

Flush the anesthesia machine per manufacturer recommendations and change out the CO_2 absorbent to get all the molecules of anesthesia vapor out of the machine. Another option is to place a specialized filter on the inspiratory and expiratory arms of the anesthesia machine which does not allow anesthesia vapor to enter the breathing circuit.

Utilize a total intravenous anesthetic (TIVA) so that no volatile anesthetics and/or succinylcholine is given. For TIVA, the most common medication used is propofol plus opioid (fentanyl or morphine) or other hypnotic agents such as midazolam, dexmedetomidine, and N2O (N2O and O2 are perfectly safe to use even in known MH cases).

Treatment

Should you have a patient with suspected MH, do the following:

1. Stop the volatile anesthetic and succinylcholine
2. Disconnect from anesthesia machine
3. Get help
4. Notify the surgeon to finish the surgery as quickly as possible
5. If the surgery ending will be prolonged, start a TIVA
6. Get the MH cart so you can start treatment with dantroline

   - Dantrolene is very hard to reconstitute. Get as much help in the room to help mix the dantrolene into solution.
   - 2.5 mg/kg rapidly IV through large-bore IV

7. Obtain an arterial line to assess need for treatment:

   - Metabolic acidosis treatment:
     - hyperventilate the patient
     - give bicarbonate
   - Hyperkalemia:
     - give insulin and glucose to drive the potassium into the cells

8. Treat dysrhythmias

   - treat acidosis
   - treat hyperkalemia
   - standard ACLS protocols

9. Cool the patient
   - gastric lavage with ice water
   - bladder lavage with ice water
   - ice packs to head, axilla, and exposed body

Continue to Follow

1. core temperature
2. ETCO2
3. laboratory studies:
   - blood gasses
   - electrolytes,
   - creatine kinase (CK)
   - serum myoglobin
   - coagulation studies
4. urine output and color

32. On Your Own for the First Time

At some point during your training, you will be left by yourself in the OR. When you are prepared to handle common problems, you can alleviate some of your anxiety. Anesthesia looks easy when you anticipate issues and proactively fix the issue before it becomes a bigger problem. <u>When you have to react to problems, you need to stay calm and make all your movements count.</u> Having an organized mind and organized equipment will help.

If you are running into problems, call your attending/preceptor sooner rather than later. There is no harm in calling your attending/preceptor, working at fixing the problem, and then having it fixed before they enter the room.

For each case, have the following readily available:

1. Your attending's pager number / cell phone number
   - What is the easiest way to get help?
2. How to contact an anesthesia tech
   - To help you get supplies
3. The name of your circulator RN in your OR
   - To help you get your attending in the room quickly

Before your attending leaves the room:

Make sure you understand the goals of your anesthetic plan. For general anesthesia, this means pain control, hypnosis, paralysis, possible regional anesthesia, and hemodynamic goals.

One of the hemodynamic goals of most anesthetics is to keep the heart rate and blood pressure within 20% of preoperative values. For more critical patients, it may mean keeping them within 10% of preoperative values. You may need to utilize your volatile anesthesia, opioids, induction agents, and vasoactive drugs to make this happen.

General Advice

If you are uncomfortable with a situation, contact your attending/preceptor to get their input.

Do not get focused on one vital sign and forget the others. You need to treat the patient as a whole system. For example, an isolated heart rate recording does not mean much without a blood pressure measurement to go with it. If you start treating the heart rate without paying attention to the blood pressure, you may come to the wrong conclusion.

The guidelines below are just that—guidelines. You should start to take steps to figure out the solution to issues while your attending/ preceptor is coming back to the room.

The operating room is a dynamic environment. Learning how to anticipate issues before they become real problems is part of the art and science of anesthesiology. What separates the mediocre anesthetist from the great anesthetist is learning how to anticipate issues and deal with them before they become problems. With experience, you will gain muscle memory and skill and some of these processes will become second nature to you.

When a situation does occur:

1. Stay calm.
    - Start working on a solution to the problem.
    - You might be able to fix it on your own before your attending/preceptor comes into the room.

2. Contact your attending early on in the problem.

- They expect phone calls/pages.
- They want to know about issues before they become big problems.
- It is better to get help before things go really bad.
- As you progress in your training, you will be calling your attending/preceptor less often because you will be able to manage most situations on your own.

3. If it is something really bad, alert the surgeon and the circulating RN.

When your attending/preceptor comes to the room.

Think through what you saw and what you did. Articulate to your attending/preceptor the sequence of events so that they can help you learn from the event. Own up to what happened and what you did. If you make a mistake, own up to it so that you and your staff can stabilize the patient and move on.

Decreased SpO2

A SpO2 that is downtrending, either slowly or quickly, is a problem. You need to really be working quickly as the SpO2 approaches 92%. There is about a 20–30 second difference between the O2 delivery to the lung and the SpO2 on the finger.

↓ SpO2 Checklist

- Contact your attending/preceptor
- Check the EtCO2
  - Has the waveform changed? Is it still present?
  - Did the patient stop breathing?
  - Is the patient still connected to the anesthesia machine?
    - Visually check to make sure the breathing circuit has not become disconnected at any point.
    - Most common place for a disconnect is at Y adaptor at the connection to the ETT.
- Is the pulse oximeter still attached to the patient?
- Place the patient on 100% O2.
- Switch machine to manually ventilate the patient.
  - Compliance of the lungs
    - Is the patient having a bronchospasm?
- Check breath sounds
  - Are they equal?

- If they are only heard on one side, then consider either:
    1. Right main stem intubation (most likely — simply pull the ETT back until bilateral breath sounds are heard).
    2. Pneumothorax (less likely — the patient would need a chest tube to fix this issue).

▫ Consider manually giving larger breaths to "recruit" alveoli that may be partially collapsed.

▫ Consider suctioning the ETT if the peak inspiratory pressure (PIP) is high.

▫ If still having issues, make sure you get your attending involved.

Decreased EtCO2

Besides HR, the EtCO2 is one of the most responsive monitors that you have at your disposal. It can alert you to issues before they become problems. The decrease or absence of EtCO2 can be as simple as a circuit disconnect, or it may be heralding a huge problem.

↓ EtCO2 Checklist:

- ▫ Consider contacting your attending/preceptor
- ▫ Make sure the EtCO2 monitor is not "auto zeroing"
    - Usually there will be a message on the monitor when it does this.
- ▫ Look for movement of
    - the ventilator bag (if the patient is breathing spontaneously) or
    - the ventilator bellows (if the patient is on the ventilator).
- ▫ Is the patient still connected to the anesthesia machine?
- ▫ Are there problems with the CO2 detector?
    - ▫ Is the sample line kinked or partially disconnected?
    - ▫ Is the "water trap" filled with moisture, or does it need to be replaced?
- ▫ Switch machine to manually ventilate the patient.

- ▫ Check breath sounds
  - • Can you give good tidal volumes?
  - • Are they equal?
  - • If they are only heard on one side, then consider either:
- • Check breath sounds (continued)
  - • Right main stem intubation (most likely—simply pull the ETT back until bilateral breath sounds are heard).
  - • Pneumothorax (less likely—the patient would need a chest tube to fix this issue).
- ▫ Compliance of the lungs
  - • Possible bronchospasm?
- ▫ Is there a leak in the system?
  - ▫ A common leak is a ruptured or inadequately inflated ETT balloon.
  - ▫ If the leak is not on the patient side, is there a leak in the machine?
- ▫ Call the anesthesia tech to help you troubleshoot the machine.
- ▫ Is the patient being over ventilated?
  - ▫ Check the tidal volumes and respiratory rate
    - • You might be hyperventilating the patient.
- ▫ Check the vital signs
  - ▫ Is the BP low?
  - ▫ Is the HR low or high?
  - ▫ ↓Cardiac output or a pulmonary embolism can cause a ↓ EtCO2 as well.

Increased EtCO2

The most common cause of an increase in EtCO2 is under ventilation. The most dire cause of increase in EtCO2 is malignant hyperthermia (MH).

↑ **EtCO2 Checklist:**

- Consider contacting your attending/preceptor.
- Is the patient being under ventilated?
    - Check the tidal volumes and respiratory rate.
    - What is your peak inspiratory pressure (PIP)?
- Is the patient breathing spontaneously?
    - Then consider assisting to correct the hypoventilation.
- Malignant hyperthermia (MH)!
    - Do the other vital signs indicate MH?
        - Tachycardia?
        - Hypertension?
        - Masseter muscle spasm?
        - Obtain an ABG to confirm/disprove the diagnosis.

Increased Peak Inspiratory Pressures (PIP)

This is seen when the patient is on the ventilator and your "high peak inspiratory pressure" alarm sounds.

↑ PIP Checklist:

- Consider contacting your attending/preceptor.
- Is the patient "light" and "fighting" the ventilator?
  - Does the patient need more anesthetic?
    - If so, consider giving a bolus of opioid or propofol? Deepen gas?
- Does the patient also need more muscle relaxant?
  - After the patient has had his or her anesthetic deepened, then check twitches and give more relaxant.
- Switch machine to manually ventilate the patient.
  - Check breath sounds
    - Are they equal or only heard on right side? (right main stem)
    - Is the patient developing a pneumothorax? (breath sounds more distant on one side vs. the other)
  - Compliance of the lungs—possible bronchospasm?
- Is the ETT or breathing circuit kinked or obstructed?
  - Consider suctioning the ETT
- In laparoscopic cases, is the abdominal pressure too high?

Heart Rate and Blood Pressure Issues

HR recordings and BP measurements are tightly coupled together. As you work through issues with heart rate and blood pressure, remember the formula from chapter 12.

BP = CO X SVR

BP = (HR x SV) x SVR

This will help you come up with a working diagnosis to fix issues. Think to yourself, "How are the HR and BP related?"

- Is the HR reflexively high because of a low BP?

- Is the BP low because of a low HR?

- Are the BP and HR both elevated because the patient is in pain or does not have enough anesthesia?

The Automatic BP Cuff

On the automatic BP cuff, the mean arterial pressure (MAP) is the most accurate number because it is actually measured (as the automatic BP cuff inflates, and subsequently deflates, the point at which blood flow through the artery is at maximal oscillation is the recorded MAP). The systolic and diastolic pressures are calculated from the MAP by using an algorithm. The MAP is the most accurate recording tool for noninvasive BP measurements.

Always obtain a baseline BP before you induce the patient. This gives you a frame of reference for the rest of the case. Doing this also checks your machine to make sure the BP cuff is the right size and the machine is working.

During the case, if the BP cuff is continually inflating/deflating and not giving you a BP reading, this can be caused by several issues:

1. The BP is very high and the BP cuff is having a hard time figuring out the range.
2. The BP is very low and the BP cuff cannot obtain a reading.
3. There is a leak in the BP cuff or tubing.
4. There is a malfunction in the BP component of the machine.
5. The BP mode might be set improperly (having the adult mode selected when checking the BP of a neonate).

If the BP cuff is continually cycling, check a pulse to make sure the patient's BP is not very low or high. Most commonly, if the BP cuff is not providing you with a BP reading, then the patient's BP is very low and you need to start treating it immediately.

The Invasive BP Monitor: The Arterial Line

When you are using an arterial line (A-line), the systolic and diastolic pressures are actually measured. It is the MAP that is calculated from these two numbers with an A-line.

Five practical things to remember about arterial lines:

1. Make sure you know the transducer for the A-line is placed at the level of the heart (for general cases) or at the level of the external auditory canal (for neurosurgical cases).

    - If the transducer is too low compared to the patient, the BP will be artificially high.

- If the transducer is too high compared to the patient, the BP will be artificially low.
- Every time you change the height of the bed, make sure the transducer is at the correct height.

2. A-lines are used for two things:
   - invasive monitoring of the BP
   - obtaining blood samples

3. Make sure the A-line is well labeled so that you don't accidentally put IV medications in them.
   - Some IV medications placed in an artery can cause severe vasoconstriction and destroy blood flow to the hand — the patient would lose his or her hand.

4. Some institutions use a low dose heparin solution for the A-line fluid.
   - If you draw back on the A-line to obtain labs, make sure you completely flush the blood from the A-line tubing so that you don't get a clot in the tubing from the blood.
   - When you flush arterial lines, make sure there is no air in the system that would get flushed into the artery and potentially cause arterial blockage.

5. We most commonly place the A-line in the radial artery on the patient's non-dominate hand.
   - There are two main blood supplies to the hand: the radial artery and the ulnar

artery. The ulnar artery is larger and provides more blood supply to the hand than the radial artery. Historically, the radial artery was used for arterial lines so that if the radial artery was compromised, the blood would still be supplied to the hand by the ulnar artery.

• If the one of the arteries on one hand is compromised, then it is generally recommended to not attempt the A-line on the other artery.

• Ultrasound has somewhat changed the practice of arterial line placement; now A-lines can be placed under direct visualization.

• Besides the radial artery, we can also use the brachial, axillary, femoral, dorsal pedal, or posterior tibial artery.

↑ HR and ↓ BP

If this is your first BP in the OR, make sure the BP cuff is not too big for the patient.

❏ If the BP is low, or the BP cuff continues to cycle and will not give you a blood pressure, check a pulse.

   ❏ If strong, consider you may be dealing with a very high BP (see below).

   ❏ If pulse is weak, consider a very low BP and treat with ephedrine or epinephrine.

   ❏ If pulse is unattainable, start CPR.

   ❏ If BP ↓, consider turning down the anesthesia volatile.

      • Realize you could potentially be increasing the risk of recall.

❏ If BP ↓ even after decreasing volatile,

   • consider IV fluid boluses

   • consider giving a bolus of phenylephrine (typically start with 50 mcg in an adult patient).

↑ HR and ↑ BP

If this is your first BP in the OR, make sure the BP cuff is not too small for the patient.

❑ Deepen the anesthesia with opioid, volatile, or propofol.

❑ If the BP and HR are unresponsive to deepening anesthesia,

• get your attending in the room and get esmolol ready;

• consider esmolol, labetalol, or metoprolol; and

• check the EtCO2 — if it is rising as well, think MH.

❑ Causes of ↑ BP and ↑ HR not responsive to deepening anesthesia include

❑ ETT on the tracheal carina,

❑ tourniquet pain (when a tourniquet is placed on the patient), and

❑ malignant hyperthermia (MH).

↓ HR and ↓ BP

If this is your first BP in the OR, make sure the BP cuff is not too big for the patient.

- If the BP is low, or the BP cuff continues to cycle and will not give you a blood pressure, check a pulse.
    - If strong, consider you may be dealing with a very high BP (see below).
    - If pulse is weak, consider a very low BP and treat with ephedrine or epinephrine.
    - If pulse is unattainable, start CPR.
    - If low, consider turning down the anesthesia volatile.
        - Realize you could potentially be increasing the risk of recall under anesthesia.
        - The patient remembers feeling or hearing things in the operating room or is awake during the procedure.
- For adult patients consider
    - glycopyrrolate 0.2–0.4 mg (1 to 2 ml)
    - ephedrine 5–10 mg (1 to 2 ml)
- If the HR is trending toward asystole in the adult patient,
    - consider epinephrine (10 mcg/kg)

↓ HR and ↑ BP

If this is your first BP in the OR, make sure the BP cuff is not too small for the patient.

- If using an arterial line, cycle the noninvasive BP cuff and make sure the A-line transducer is at the proper level.
- If the HR is still low, wait for your attending.
    - This can be a very bad sign: increased intracranial pressure (ICP).
- ❏ If ↑ ICP is suspected,
    - ❏ put patient on 100% O2 and
    - ❏ start hyperventilating the patient;
    - ❏ you may need to give mannitol.
- ❏ If ↑ ICP is not suspected,
    - ❏ you need to give hydralazine, nitroglycerine, or sodium nitroprusside.

The Patient Moves During Surgery

There can be a number of reasons why a patient moves during surgery.

The patient may not have enough anesthesia and may be responding to surgery (it may also be that the BP cuff is inflating and the surgeon feels the movement).

Sometimes you can tell the patient is getting "light" with either an increase in BP or HR before the patient moves.

Movement under anesthesia does not necessarily mean that the patient will remember surgery, but you need to stay calm and move quickly. During some surgeries, patient movement can be frustrating to the surgeon. In other cases, patient movement can be dangerous or catastrophic.

Patient Movement Checklist:

- ☐ Check vital signs to make sure the patient is stable.
- ☐ Make sure the patient is not sliding off the table or changing positions on the bed.
- ☐ Does the patient need more anesthetic?
    - ☐ Give a bolus of opioid or "dial up" the anesthesia vapor.
        - ☐ If the patient is hemodynamically stable, consider giving 0.5–1 mg/kg of propofol to deepen.
- ☐ Does the patient also need more muscle relaxant?
    - After the patient has been deepened, check for twitches and give more relaxant.
        - Just giving muscle relaxants to stop patient movement may increase the risk of awareness under anesthesia.
        - Always deepen the anesthetic first, and then paralyze if necessary.
        - If the patient's HR/BP will not tolerate more anesthesia, then consider using pressors to increase the HR or BP so that you can increase the anesthesia.

33. Your Pregnancy and Your Anesthesia / Airway Rotation

Adding to your family can be an exciting time in your life. As with many exciting things in life, there can also be some anxiety. Always check with your personal obstetrician regarding your exposure to the OR environment and any special precautions you need to take. The following are general guidelines and you should also defer to your personal obstetrician for their recommendations.

The benefits of being in the OR include participating in an anesthesia observation, working with real patients in an airway rotation, or doing an anesthesia rotation to see what anesthesiology is all about. There are some risks, however.

The operating room can be a dangerous environment. There are sharp instruments and the possibility of infectious disease transmission as well as exposure to radiation and potential teratogenic medications. These can present a number of potential challenges for the pregnant trainee during your anesthesia rotation.

Check with the administrators of the institution where you will be doing your observation/rotation to see if they have any policies or procedures regarding pregnant trainees. It is always best to keep them in the loop. The following is a short list of considerations for you on your observation/rotation.

Staying Hydrated

It is common practice for anesthesia students/residents (and attendings working by themselves) to be relatively dehydrated. We don't want to be in the middle of a case and have to go to the bathroom, and we can't drink fluids during cases. With longer cases in particular, we tend to be more dehydrated than someone who has free access to oral fluids and a bathroom. Talk with your staff. We understand that pregnant students/residents have to urinate more as they progress in their pregnancy. Stay hydrated and communicate with your faculty when you need to go to the bathroom. Getting dehydrated and going into premature contractions would not be good.

Disease Transmission

There are times when you will be taking care of patients who have a contagious disease. Always wear gloves, face mask, and eye shields. Many contagious diseases are spread through the blood. You may consider getting re-fitted for your tuberculosis face mask because your face shape may change with the changes in hormones within your body. It would be preferable to avoid patients with active TB, or at the very least, limit your exposure with TB specific masks. Wash your hands frequently, and take even more care when handling needles and sharp instruments.

Radiation Exposure

Radiation exposure is the one thing that has been consistently shown to be a risk for the pregnant trainee and her fetus as a teratogen. This is perhaps the most obvious risk and easiest to avoid. Request that you are not placed in anesthesia locations with high radiation exposure.

Places where radiation exposure is common include the following:

1. Orthopedics rooms
    - Surgical rooms
    - Casting rooms
2. Fluoroscopy rooms
    - Cath lab
    - Interventional radiology
3. Dental rooms due to dental x-rays.
4. Rooms where central lines are placed
    - Fluoroscopy is commonly used in these rooms.

If you are assigned to one of these rooms:

1. Limit your exposure
    - Try to switch out of the room if radiation is going to be used.
    - Step outside the room during x-ray use, if possible.

2. Protect yourself
   1. Use a full wraparound gown.
      - In anesthesia, it is very difficult to keep your front side facing the radiation source at all times.
   2. Along with the full wraparound lead gown, use a standing lead shield between you and the radiation source.
3. Put some distance between you and the radiation source.
   - The farther away you are from the radiation source, the less the exposure.
   - Radiation reduces significantly with distance from the radiation source.

Limit Your Exposure to Nitrous Oxide (N2O)

N_2O has also been shown to be a teratogen. High levels of exposure to N_2O have been shown to cause spontaneous abortions in dental assistants who have side exposure to N_2O in environments without a scavenging system. In the anesthesia literature, a report from the United Kingdom (UK) showed that "the incidence of infertility, spontaneous abortion and children with congenital abnormalities in female anesthesiologists to be the same as that in other physicians."

Although this is believed to be true, we would still recommend that you limit your exposure.

1. Avoid using N2O during the anesthetic.
2. With all anesthetics, whether or not you are using N2O, use good waste gas management skills:

- Use a good tight mask seal when doing mask inductions and when manually ventilating patients.

- When the breath circuit is not directly attached to the patient (mask off the face or circuit disconnected from the ETT or LMA), turn off the gas flow.

- Make sure the scavenging system is working properly on your anesthesia machine.

Limit Your Exposure to Methyl Methacrylate

Methyl methacrylate is the bone cement used by orthopedic surgeons for joint replacements. Although radiation exposure in the orthopedic rooms brings risk to you and your fetus, so does bone cement. When the cement is prepared for placement in the patient, to secure the point, the exothermic process releases a pungent smell that may potentially be harmful to an unborn baby. Ask either to not be in these types of surgeries or to have someone care for the patient during that part of the surgery.

Recognize / Limit Stress

There are two types of stress that you will encounter in the operating room: physical and emotional. Although it is difficult to avoid these situations in anesthesiology, recognize that stress is a job hazard of anesthesiology. Do what you can to limit the physical stress (get good sleep, rest when you can, don't stand when you can sit) and the emotional stress (know your patients well, have a good anesthesia plan in place, and have a well prepared room/equipment).

34. Anesthesia Resources

There are a variety of different resources available for anesthesia trainees at all levels of training — from anesthesia technologists to anesthesiology fellows. To make it easy for you to find the resources I personally recommend, I have put together an organized list for you at AnesthesiaMadeEasy.com. On this web page, you will find links to anesthesia resources, reviews of anesthesia books, and recommendations of other types of books you may be interested in. My two favorite starting books are *Morgan and Mikhail's Clinical Anesthesiology* (5th edition) and *Basics of Anesthesia: Expert Consult — Online and Print* (6th edition).

Getting into Anesthesia Residency

To keep this book at a reasonable size, I have given you the basics of getting the most from your anesthesia rotation. I do offer a FREE e-book on AnesthesiaMadeEasy.com — *Getting Into Anesthesiology* — that is an insider's guide to getting into anesthesiology residency for medical school students and residents who change specialties. The 25-page PDF discusses what an anesthesiologist's career is like, how to see if anesthesiology is the career for you, how to prepare your application, and how to get the most from your limited number of elective rotations in medical school.

Epilogue

I hope you enjoyed this book, and I want to encourage you to continue your anesthesia training and check out the resources that I have for you on my website www.AnesthesiaMadeEasy.com.

The challenge in writing a book such as this is to provide enough information to be helpful and not so much information that the reader is overwhelmed (there are plenty of overwhelming anesthesiology texts available). Perhaps there are areas that would have been helpful for you that I should have included in the book.

Is there something I missed? I would love to hear from you. Please send me an e-mail at jeff@TwoPugsPublishing.com

Also, if you enjoyed the book, I would really appreciate it if you would please go to amazon.com and write a review.

Best Regards,
Jeff Steiner, DO, MBA

About the Author

Dr. Steiner works as a Pediatric Anesthesiologist in Dallas, Texas, and is the program director for the Pediatric Anesthesiology Fellowship Program at his institution. Before starting medical school, he worked as a full-time paramedic after completing college and held the Emergency Medical Technician–Tactical (EMT-T) certification for support of Special Weapons and Tactics (SWAT) teams. He graduated medical school from Texas College of Osteopathic Medicine and continued his training at UT Southwestern Medical Center.

During his residency training in anesthesiology, he edited *The Acute Pain Manual*, which was a survival guide for residents while on the acute pain service and developed "Vapor Camp," a one month introduction for anesthesiology interns to prepare them for the operating room. Dr. Steiner was chief resident his senior year. For the last eight years, he has been a member of Outcomes Research Consortium, which is an international research group based out of the Cleveland Clinic.

Dr. Steiner's research interests include pediatric airway management, respiratory monitoring, and residents' medical school debt management. And he is author of the book *The Physician's Guide to Personal Finance: The Review Book for the Class You Never Had in Medical School.*

Dr. Steiner is currently double boarded in anesthesiology and pediatric anesthesiology and continues to teach anesthesiologists assistant students, residents, fellows, and airway rotators in the art and science of pediatric anesthesiology.

Common Abbreviations

AA - anesthesiologist assistant

ABG - arterial blood gas

ASA – American Society of Anesthesiologists

BP – blood pressure

CO2 – carbon dioxide

CRNA - certified registered nurse anesthetist

ECG - electrocardiogram (some call it an EKG - German spelling)

EMLA – eutectic mixture of local anesthetics

EtCO2 - end tidal carbon dioxide that is expelled from the patient

ETT – endotracheal tube

FiO2 – fraction of inspired oxygen (expressed as a decimal, not a percentage.)

HR – heart rate

ICU – intensive care unit

IV - intravenous

kg – kilogram

LA – local anesthetic

MAC – minimum alveolar concentration

mcg - micrograms

mg – milligrams

ml – milliliter (1 ml = 1 cc)

N2O – nitrous oxide

NPO – nothing by mouth (nil per os)

OR – operating room

PACU – post-anesthesia care unit (aka recovery room)

PCA – patient controlled analgesia

PCO2 - carbon dioxide partial pressure

PEEP – positive end-expiratory pressure

PIP - peak inspiratory pressure

PO - by mouth (per os)
PRN – as needed
RSI - rapid sequence induction

References

Chapter 4

ASA Taskforce on Sedation and Analgesia by Non-Anesthesiologists "Practice Guidelines for Sedation and Analgesia by Non-Anesthesiologists." *Anesthesiology* 2002; 96: 1004–17. American Society of Anesthesiologists, Inc. Lippincott Williams & Wilkins, Inc.

Chapter 6–16

Flood, Rathmell, and Shafer, MD. *Stoelting's Pharmacology and Physiology in Anesthetic Practice. Fifth edition* Published by Lippincott Williams & Wilkins: 2014

Levine, Wilton C., MD, et al. *Clinical Anesthesia Procedures of the Massachusetts General Hospital. Eighth edition* Published by Lippincott Williams & Wilkins: 2010

Whalen, Karen (PharmD BCPS). *Lippincott Illustrated Reviews: Pharmacology Sixth edition.* Published by Lippincott Williams & Wilkins: 2014

Chapter 17

Gan et al. 2014. "Consensus Guidelines for the Management of Postoperative Nausea and Vomiting." *Anesthesia & Analgesia* 118(1):85–113.

Chapter 19

STOP - BANG reference.

Chung, F. et al. 2008. "A Tool to Screen Patients for Obstructive Sleep Apnea." *Anesthesiology* 108:812–21. American Society of Anesthesiologists, Inc. Lippincott Williams & Wilkins, Inc.

Chapter 23

Recommendations for Pre-Anesthesia Checkout Procedures (2008). Accessed March 1, 2015. www.asahq.org

Chapter 25

Koh et al. 2002. "Modified Cormack-Lehane Scale: The Modified Cormack-Lehane Score for the Grading of Direct Laryngoscopy: Evaluation in the Asian Population." *Anaesthesia and Intensive Care* 30(1):48–51.

Chapter 26

Litman Elsevier, R., editor *Pediatric Anesthesia: The Requisites in Anesthesiology*. Published by Mosby 2004. (Unfortunately … out of print. ☹)

Chapter 32

Malignant Hyperthermia Association of the United States http://www.mhaus.org/ Accessed March 1, 2015.

Chapter 34

Miller et al. *Miller's Anesthesia Eidth edition. Page 3055* Published by Saunders 2014

My Notes

My Notes

My Notes

Made in the USA
Middletown, DE
03 June 2024

55211589R00102